BY-PASS

By the same author:
Zig Zag to Armageddon

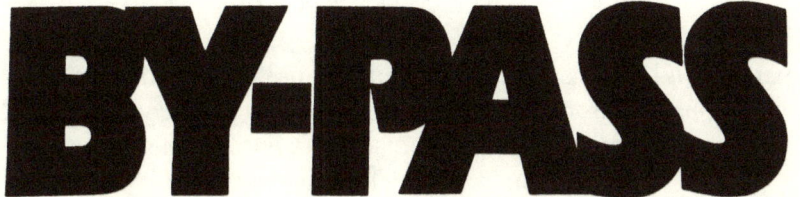

Tony Foster

Authors Choice Press

San Jose New York Lincoln Shanghai

By-Pass

Authors Choice Press
an imprint of iUniverse.com, Inc.

For information address:
iUniverse.com, Inc.
620 North 48th Street, Suite 201
Lincoln, NE 68504-3467
www.iuniverse.com

The Holmes chart on page 166 reprinted from *Stressful Life Events—Their Nature and Effects* by B.S. Dohrenwend and Bruce Philip Dohrenwend (1974) with permission from John Wiley and Sons, Inc., N.Y.

Originally published by Methuen

ISBN: 0-595-13749-0

Printed in the United States of America

Dedicated to every coronary conqueror who has heard the soft, enticing rustle of angel feathers and realized that life is sweet.

"A thousand times I have heard men tell
That there is joy in Heaven and Pain in Hell
And I accord right well that it is so.
And yet indeed full well myself I know
That there is not a man in this countrie
That either has in Heaven or Hell y'be."

"The Chaunteclere," from
The Canterbury Tales by
Geoffrey Chaucer, 1400

"The heart alone of all viscera has reached
the limits set by nature to surgery. No new
method and no new technique can overcome
the natural obstacles surrounding a wound of
the heart."

Sir Stephen Paget, Surgeon
London, England, 1896

Contents

For hours it has fought the treacherous channels, squirming through soft, moist darkness, over rifts, shoals, past swirling eddies. Tens of thousands have fallen by the wayside in this titanic struggle. Yet still it moves, slowly, steadily ahead to that ultimate prize.

Finally, close to exhaustion, the blunt head nudges a mucous surface. One last wriggle to penetrate and its journey ends.

The trigger of life is gathered into the ovum. DNA molecules spin, merging program codes defining this new unique being *that* they will build between them.

Cells divide, again, again, and again. Ten million years of man's ascent from the ocean's slime to be compressed into two hundred and eighty days.

Within minutes the gelatinous embryo starts pulsating. The first miniscule beat of what will grow into a human heart.

Prologue

Kingston, Canada
2 July 1980

After psyching yourself into accepting the inevitable, it is the waiting that finally gets to you. What laughing deity divided life into a series of waits? Waiting to be born, to walk, talk, learn. Waiting for unfulfilled hopes, disasters, waiting to grow old. Then waiting to die. Will I die today? Anything is possible.

On the tenth floor of Kingston General Hospital five gurneys are parked in the holding room, each awaiting a green light from the surgeon that its operating room is ready and waiting. I lie on one of the five. My appointment is for 8:00 A.M. I'm early. So I wait.

Each patient's hospital records are clipped to the cover wrapping their feet. Too far to reach, too far to read. Mine says CORONARY BY-PASS, DR. T. SALERNO. I read it in the elevator on the way up. My eyes are fine. It's my heart that is giving me troubles.

For forty-seven years it pumped millions of gallons of blood through miles of arteries and veins. Then it failed. Myocardial infarct are the buzz words. To my layman's ear it still sounds nebulous. Why can't they call it a heart attack? Physicians and lawyers are brothers in dissembling the obvious.

Lying next to me, a thin old woman with wrinkled leather face, whiskered forelip, and large, luminous eyes nods agreeably.

"Lovely morning."

1

We could have been sharing the sidewalk in front of a bus stop. Her voice is young and musical. She is quite right. Beyond the institutional green there is a lovely July morning. I awoke early to inspect it from my hospital window and sat drinking in its beauty in much the same way that a condemned man sucks that last cigarette while the firing squad fidgets with embarrassment.

What a lovely day to die! Summer in full bloom, the big lake calm and inviting, white clouds scampering overhead on a joyous breeze. How many other mornings have I seen like this and never noticed?

The old woman examines me myopically across the inches separating our faces.

"Anything serious?" she inquires softly.

"Coronary by-pass."

She nods again as if she had known all the time.

"I'm exploratory surgery." She sighs.

Madame Exploratory Surgery meets Mister By-Pass. How-do-you-do. There's nothing more to say. She knows I know she has cancer. I know she knows I have a dicky heart.

A nurse in green gown and face mask slips through the double-swing doors, checks the woman's records, and wheels her away. Now we are four.

Everything is green. Walls, sheets, people, complexions from the reflected overhead lights, all a hideous green. Who in hell decided green is good?

On my other side a boy stares vacantly at a spot somewhere above my head.

"Are you there?" he asks.

"I'm here."

He is six, possibly seven, with an open face etched in curiosity.

"Good, I thought they took you. I'm Kevin. I'm going to see after my operation. The doctor said so!"

Such faith. My defenses crumble after all and I begin weeping helpless tears of pity for the old woman, the blind boy, and myself. All of us on the same journey to inevitable and identical ends. Kevin has yet to learn of his mortality, while the old woman has accepted hers. I'm still trying to adjust.

They come for me. Impossible to say good-by to the others. My throat is tight, and deep within my chest that old angina andiron begins its squeezing again.

A short roll along a dim green corridor, through another door, then into bright sunlight. The brightness forces me to squint, hiding the tears.

The operating room is much smaller than I'd expected. Five gowned and masked figures are busy with chores. I've met them all but now they're unrecognizable except for the very tall, slim anesthetist who visited me late last night for a few minutes. He hums tunelessly and tosses a gloved wave in my direction as I'm rolled onto the operating table. I relax and look around.

Light flashes from the stainless-steel equipment. An array of wicked scalpels are set neatly on a folded green towel at my elbow—pans, trays, a small circular saw with tiny shiny teeth for the true hobbyist, and finally the heart-lung unit with its unobtrusive stand-by electrical system connected in case of power blackout. Everything neat and tidy and waiting to be used.

"Good morning all! I trust everybody's hands are nice and steady after a restful night's sleep?"

The strength of my voice surprises me. One of them laughs. It is enough. I know none have had a restful night's sleep for months. They are physicians for whom sleepless nights are an occupational hazard of the profession.

I.V. needles are slid into my arms. White plasma drips down clear plastic tubing from overhead glass bottles. The room feels terribly cold. It is my imagination? How can anyone's fingers maintain sufficient deftness for the delicate task ahead? Is there a thermostat they can turn up?

They gather around the table, their eyes brown, hazel, blue, and businesslike. The moment is at hand. Beyond the window I see sky, velvet blue, inviting the pilot within my soul to come tumble for a while among the clouds. Then someone pulls a switch and in a blink the darkness clamps down.

Kingston, Canada

14 January 1980

There is an elephant sitting on my chest. He's been there for hours. I can't see whether he's gray or pink but, sweet Jesus, I can feel him! Tail pressed against my breastbone, his great goddamn hams crushing out my breath. Life is trying desperately to flee my carcass while I lie imprisoned in pain.

It's nearly over. Both arms have gone dead, superfluous slabs of flesh and bone. Fingers tingle enticingly but their motor power has shut down. Involuntarily, spasms jerk my head from side to side, fighting to escape this torture. Consciousness dwells on the border of twilight waiting for the release of death.

Yet oh, how the body fights the titan of destruction, refusing to go meekly on that last great flight into the abyss. Give up! It's done, finished. Hurl life's glass to shards, then wrap the shroud and leave the party to other revelers.

Cold, dry oxygen clatters through my windpipe from a foul-smelling plastic mask held by the ambulance attendant, a young man with swarming hair and soft blue-china eyes that speak compassion and concern. He grasps my head with strong hands and murmurs sounds of animal encouragement. A siren "wheeps," pleading for right-of-way. Are the cars pulling over? Does it really matter? Will they mark me DOA—Dead On Arrival—after all?

My vital signs are radioed ahead to the hospital's emergency center; color, body temperature, respiration, heartbeat, and blood pressure.

The siren stops. Doors open. A dozen hands lift me to a gurney. Then I see people running beside my head and feet, like kids pacing a fire truck in delighted anticipation of disaster.

I float on a gauze of variable sensations, spectator instead of participant in the surrounding activity. Needles are inserted,

4

fluids injected, wires affixed, graphs traced by dancing steel pens, while above all the clamor, and sounding loud and clear, comes a steady metronomic "beep-beep-beep" from the voice of my heart.

Slowly pain recedes. The elephant floats away, leaving me so very tired and feeling completely helpless but ecstatic to be alive.

From the midst of chaos Helen appears to hold my hand and smile through swimming eyes. She doesn't speak. There is nothing to say. I doze and wake, then doze again. Then they guide her away to sign some papers. Clothes are peeled off without protest, thank-you-very-much, Mr. Foster.

"Just you lie still and let us do the work."

Gladly.

A young doctor with furry red beard and Irish accent pops from behind the curtain to introduce himself.

"You've had a heart attack," he tells me gently, lips barely moving through the red fur.

"Are you certain?"

I want to make sure this time. Two weeks before Christmas a different ambulance brought me to this same hospital, same curtained emergency room for nearly the same sort of chest pain. Not as deep, not as prolonged, not as debilitating, but agonizing nonetheless.

The diagnosis then had been severe indigestion from eating too fast. Different doctor. Different diagnosis. Like a bloody fool I accepted it.

Since then my local G.P. has been treating me with massive doses of liquid antacid which, although they did nothing for my frequent chest pains, produced what surely have been some of the longest and loudest belches on record.

"No doubt at all. You've had a myocardial infarct in the anterior coronary area."

"Please, in English, if you wouldn't mind."

"Sorry. Back of your heart, upper left side."

"Serious?"

The eyes turn evasive. Before answering he sucks at some hair under his bottom lip.

"Any heart attack is serious. Your ECG—electrocardiogram tracing—shows some damage. How much we won't know until later, after your blood count has been checked for an enzyme level."

"I see."

Which of course I don't at all, but I'm too tired to probe further and he's probably under orders not to alarm me.

"We're sending you up to the Coronary Care Unit for a few days' observation—in case complications develop." He adds his throwaway line in a tone suggesting the possibility of complications infinitesimally small and if the decision was left in his hands he'd let Helen take me home now.

"What sort of complications, doctor?"

Funny that I should ask. Does every patient entering Emergency lie acquiescent? Surely now and again one must sit up and ask what's happening to him or her.

Instead of an answer I get a smile like the horizontal tear of a fire curtain. If he has teeth, I missed them. He mumbles with the nurses, gives me a conspiratorial wink, and vanishes stage left.

Coronary Care is the end of an elevator ride on the fourth floor. Five private rooms, one wall of each a sliding glass panel that looks out to a monitor desk. There, a gimlet-eyed nurse sits watching digital displays transmitted from each heart patient inside the fishbowls. Night and day someone watches these LED heartbeats and endless fluorescent tracings, instantly alert to variations from their norm.

The first hours after an attack are the most critical. Pain comes from an inability of coronary arteries to provide oxygenated blood with which to feed the heart muscle. The pain, deep under the breastbone, is called angina pectoris.

Not all angina pains signify the onslaught of a heart attack. Usually, quite the reverse is true. But if the pain persists beyond five minutes after all physical activity is stopped, then chances are a heart attack is under way.

For some inexplicable reason most doctors are reluctant to suggest angina, preferring to regard any chest pain as torn ligaments, bruised sternum, bronchial inflammation, or indigestion. Anything but heart problems. Unfortunately, unless an ECG and blood pressure check can be done during the time that chest pains are being experienced, there is no simple way of knowing if the problem is angina pectoris or in fact simple indigestion. Only after the damage is done, the physician's diagnosis proved wrong, does the true cause of the pain become obvious.

Depending upon which coronary artery is restricted or closed to fresh blood, portions of the heart fed by this artery begin to die. The heart pumps faster and harder to compensate for the loss; other arteries take up the excess load through other narrowing passages. More pain ensues until at last stabilization takes place, the patient lies still and quiet, and the heart's demand for blood is satisfied.

But clots can form from damaged tissue, traveling the bloodstream until several hours later one or more may lodge back in the heart, causing further blockages and, ultimately, death.

Or the heart's electrical circuitry for some reason goes haywire, shuts out the brain's commands, and races into fibrillation. These rapid, irregular contractions of heart muscle can starve the entire body of fresh blood in much the same manner that a cavitating propeller or centrifugal pump produces functionless energy. Without immediate external electrical inducement to short-circuit this fibrillation command, death is mere moments away.

Or the heart can give up the fight, totally exhausted from its lifetime of titanic work and struggle. Then there is nothing that can be done.

"But in your case I foresee nothing that drastic. You're in good physical shape, still in your forties, and we're here to give you the best of care. I wish you could have met some of the basket cases we've had in here who have pulled through."

Andrew Koval is senior coronary resident physician. A tall, smooth-skinned man my age with the demeanor and features of a politician working his home hustings secure in the knowledge that his opposition doesn't stand a chance, he exudes power of the type that makes rivers run backward, old ladies swoon, and heart patients like me clutch at his words. Everything is explained in layman terms, possibilities for disaster dismissed summarily as being so remote that it's pointless to waste time discussing them.

He's bullshitting, of course, but I'm in the mood to be bullshitted, needing desperately to believe in my survival. Two hours ago I faced death in a sea of pain. Now I face life in an ocean of optimism provided by Dr. Koval and his entourage of interns, nurses, and junior resident. I'm overwhelmed by the attention.

They tap, probe, listen, muse, discuss their findings, and nod knowingly. A nurse elbows her way bedside with a hotdog vendor's tray cluttered with glass test tubes. Expertly, she stabs an arm vein and begins taking blood, oblivious to the others.

"Are you feeling any pain now?" an intern asks.

"A dull ache. But no pain—that's gone."

"Can you describe your pain, what it was like? Steady pain or rising and falling with intensity?"

I look to Koval for help. He awards an encouraging smile. For a minute or two I try explaining the elephant. They nod like people who have heard the punch line to the joke before at a different party, different bedside. They know all about my elephant.

"We're going to put you on a beta-block tablet. Inderal, twenty milligrams every eight hours to start. It does all sorts of good things for your heart. Provides more oxygenated blood, lowers your pulse rate and blood pressure, lets your heart relax while it repairs itself."

The stuff sounds omnipotent. I can hardly wait for my first pill to arrive. At my elbow the vampire finishes filling a half-dozen vacuum tubes, loads everything onto her hotdog tray, and departs with a perfunctory smile of thanks.

Another technician appears at the doorway to my fishbowl, a wisp of a girl peeking from behind a giant robot. The infernal machine whines to a stop.

"Mr. Foster?"

Are we to be introduced or engorged? The others scramble from the robot's path. It whines alongside my bed, its huge, glaring eye inches from my head. The girl checks my hospital wristband in case I've been lying to her, then says, "X-ray," and proceeds to work.

How many REMs will the machine use of my body's bank balance? Roentgen Equivalent Man, REM for short, is the measure of radiation absorbed by the human body. It is accumulative in its damage and can, in overdoses, cause cancer and birth defects. But then so can toothpaste if you're silly enough to swallow a few tubes of the stuff. Still, I notice that the doctors and nurses stand well back from the unit's cyclopic eye when the technician tells me to take a deep breath ... and ... hold it!

Then, as swiftly as they appeared, everyone leaves; the robot, its tiny driver, nurses, interns, resident, and the Mighty Koval, my security beacon.

They let Helen in for a few minutes. Her movements are jerky, a piano-wire tautness to every lip and cheek muscle, pale hands, and waxen face with startled eyes. How I adore her. So much to bear for so long; now this.

"I'm fine. The doctor says I'll be as good as new. Look at all the wires and electronics, will you? I'll bet if I fart somewhere a bell will ring, bringing a squad of nurses rushing out of the woodwork."

She smiles and squeezes my hand even though it's not much of a joke. An intern appears, holding a clipboard, and wants to ask a million questions. Helen promises to come back in the afternoon.

Is it still only morning?

"Yes, doctor, I am allergic to penicillin, caffeine, and tetracycline. No, there is no history of heart problems in my family. Parents and grandparents all died very early of cancer or very late of old age. Ditto on TB and diabetes, no family history."

Heredity is the most serious aspect to coronary insufficiencies. Like those genes that produce a parent's facial characteristics, hair color and texture, or a grandparent's superb constitution, other genes are passed down with serious deficiencies. In midlife, when the body's ability to replace its cellular structures begins to slow and the aging process starts, these deficiencies appear. Weak kidneys, liver ailments, pancreas and stomach problems, in many cases can be traced directly through family antecedents.

After eliminating the heredity angle he switches saddles. "Do you smoke?"

"Every day for thirty-two years. But I quit this morning."

"About time, I'd say."

Next to heredity, smoking is the worst abuse that can be given the heart. Did I realize this? Shamefaced, I mumble something suitably contrite, but he isn't about to let the matter drop. This kid is fresh from university medical school, his brain vibrating with the very latest gen.

"Beyond clogging your lungs with black sticky goo, developing emphysema and progressive cancer, there is the matter of starving your body's oxygen requirements. Do you realize that every time you puff one of those filthy cigarettes you're inhaling poisonous carbon monoxide gas that's going straight into your blood stream? Result: up goes your blood pressure and heart rate. In long-term damage you're hastening hardening of the arteries. And you've been doing this for over thirty years. Madness!"

His eyes shine with evangelical zeal. I'm convinced, brother. A true believer since early this morning when my elephant turned up to squat. But I do wish this guy would get on with his questions so that I can get to sleep. My mind is weary.

In succession I'm awakened for pills, "thank you," lunch, "no thank you, I'm not hungry," further temperature and pressure checks, and more blood from the hotdog lady. I can't imagine what she's doing with it all. Even the X-ray robot glides back for a replay. Apparently my chest is a shade too wide for the negative. They need a photograph of the missing part. Finally, all is quiet, the door slides shut, and I am left in peace.

My room is bright and airy, the chrome-covered oxygen equipment and wall fittings appear new and well maintained.

The furnishings are modern and beautifully clean. Even the crucifix hanging high against the wall above my bed is of recent casting. It and the hospital's name, Hotel Dieu—God's Hotel— are the only visible evidence or acknowledgment of its religious origins.

Below my window and across the street is a former residence of Sir John A. MacDonald, Canada's first prime minister. History outside my windowpane. It's a stone house, three stories, built in simple rectangular symmetry with beautiful dormers. I've never visited the place. Why is it that we never bother to inspect the wonders in our own back yards?

A few years ago in Rio de Janeiro I took a cable car to the top of Sugarloaf Mountain. My Brazilian partner complained about this waste of time. All his life he'd lived in Rio and never climbed the Sugarloaf until I dragged him to its summit. I've forgotten now whether he enjoyed the trip or that spectacular view of the city and its gleaming white sandy beaches, but when he came north to visit me the following year the first place I had to drive him was to Niagara Falls.

"But, Marcos, it's only water rushing over a cliff to splash into a rainbow!"

"Philistine!" he snarled. "Have you no soul?"

Lying in bed, grazing in my field of thoughts, I try to come to terms with my mortality. Until now wars, revolutions, accidents, or hospitals claimed the other poor sods, never me. The immortality of optimism, watching the rest of the world succumb while death brushes past without so much as a nod or fleeting whisper in my direction.

It's the reason teenagers make the best soldiers. Filled with the courage of blind ignorance of odds and statistics, they cannot conceive of their own destruction until it is too late to leave the game of war. Then, suddenly, they are too old to care.

Helen returns and sits quietly watching me. In sleep I can feel her eyes.

"Hullo, been here long?"

"A few minutes. I didn't want to disturb you."

"How are the kids?"

"At home—fighting. They've accepted the fact that you're going to get better."

Outside, winter afternoon clouds are piled high in golden glory. The corroded metallic roof on Sir John A.'s house glints dark green at the end of a single shaft of sunlight. Snowbanks around the buildings need a fresh dusting to brush away the city's grime.

"I've been thinking."

"Yes?"

"Things will never be quite the same again."

"I know."

"Strange, isn't it? Over half a lifetime to discover that the important things were always close at hand waiting for me to reach out and touch, but I could never see them. Wealth, power, excitement, travel, success, and failure mean nothing in the long run. Why kill ourselves racing for the stars? In the end we all wind up in the same-sized box. You and the children are all I've ever really needed, a roof over our heads and food in our bellies. What a foolish journey I've been on."

"Such wisdom for a Monday afternoon."

We both laugh. We understand each other.

"So what are you going to do about it?"

"I'm going to get better! I'll start with that; the rest should be easy."

Shifts change at midnight. New faces wake me for my pills, temperature, and blood pressure. On the monitor inside my room I see my heart has slowed from its normal seventy-eight beats a minute to a lazy fifty-six. The Inderal is doing its silent work.

As the hours pass, the percentages for my survival increase. Heart rate is strong and regular. I'm wrapped in a warm cocoon of chemical contentment, secure in the knowledge that my vital signs are being watched from the desk monitor outside throughout the night. No clots nor complications for me. I drift in sleep.

Dr. Koval is back in the morning for his rounds. He breezes

in with the entourage who arrange themselves around my bed once more. He checks my pulse while eyeing the monitor.

"Still with us?"

"And intending to remain for a while."

"I never doubted it. Any chest pain?"

"No, is there supposed to be?"

I want to conform. He grins. A little-boy grin, suggesting secrets to be shared.

"There better not be any more pain. I don't permit it on this floor."

His entourage chuckle dutifully. I manage a smile.

"How much longer will I be here?"

"A few days, until you're out of the woods and feeling stronger; then we'll move you out of intensive care and down the hall with my other layabouts. Then, if you behave yourself, I'll send you home. Make it ten days in all. That suit you?"

There was a time not so long ago when heart patients were prescribed infinite amounts of rest, sentenced to a life of inactivity while their muscles—including the heart muscle—atrophied, weakened, and died. Today the universal prescription is progressive exercise once the healing process has ended. This takes about ten days to complete.

Muscles must be used in order to continue their function. The quicker this begins after discharge from hospital, the better. Rate of exercise varies among patients, depending on age, physical condition, and severity of coronary damage. The latter, in my case, cannot be determined until the end of the third day when final tabulation of blood enzymes is complete. Then I'll learn the limitations on my future existence, which can be anything from becoming a marathon runner down to a cardiac cripple seated in a wheelchair.

They poke and probe, tap and listen through their stethoscopes to my lungs, carotid arteries, and, of course, heart. A repeat of yesterday's performance but with a shade less anxiety or haste.

I do feel better. Ate some breakfast, rang for a bedpan—a foolish feeling for a grown man to be sitting on a nickel-plated toidy-seat, a thigh-length shirty draped discreetly about the ghastly business like a bell tent. But the body's functions must continue.

"Son, if y'don't eat, y'don't shit. An' if y'don't shit, y'die!" a loquacious Texan once informed me in a cookhouse down at Eagle Lake when I decided to pass on his black-eyed peas.

The Great Lord Koval gives my shoulder a pat preparatory to departing. I clasp his wrist.

"Do you know what caused it, doctor?"

"Your heart attack?" He shakes his head, "No one knows what causes heart attacks in the specific sense. If you're asking why did you have one yesterday morning, I'd say that you have an advanced case of arteriosclerosis in one of your coronary arteries that blocked the flow of blood. Quite simple. But that was the final result, not the cause. The cause started back in your youth—yours, mine, everybody's. All of us suffer from arteriosclerosis or hardening of the arteries."

He tells me how Marine doctors during the Vietnam war found cases of advanced arteriosclerosis in teen-aged combat fatalities. Young lads on the springboard to life, in the prime of physical conditioning, with coronary arteries closed 50 percent and more by a yellow waxy plaque incapable of being dissolved or absorbed by the body's mechanisms.

"They weren't born that way. With their parents' help they did it to themselves before they ever joined the Marines. Too many hotdogs, milkshakes, hamburgers, ice cream, butter, whipped cream, and, later, too many cigarettes or marijuana. If they had managed to survive Vietnam and come home, by now most would be in Coronary Care Units because of overwork, boozing, too many late nights, nagging wives, problem kids, overweight—it all takes its toll. That muscle inside our chests is an amazing little machine, considering what we do to it in our lifetime."

"But surely there's some way to prevent arteriosclerosis?"

It appears to be such a simple problem. We put men on the moon, peek at the universe's mysteries, but can't come up with something to dissolve arterial plaque?

"We're working on it, but at the moment there is only one sure way to stay clean. Never smoke, stay out of all cities, exercise eight hours every day, move to Nepal or Lapland, and live exclusively on skim milk, fresh vegetables, and fish. And above all, don't worry because tension or worry can cause heart attacks as quickly as smoking or diet."

He shrugs and gives me that little-boy grin.

"Are you ready to change your lifestyle?"

"I'm going to have to or prepare to meet my Maker—as the signs say."

Koval and his entourage swirl past the doorway, my problems forgotten already. In the next fishbowl an elderly overweight woman hovers on the brink of extinction. I heard the nurses talking to her during breakfast. She didn't want to eat, didn't want to bother anybody, just wanted to be left alone to die. Her desire to live is gone in a sputtering of fragmented memory. Arteriosclerosis has starved blood from parts of her brain, turning her senile—a slobbering, babbling eighty-year-old child of nature.

Who was it who wrote: "My candle burns at both its ends, it will not last the night. But ah my foes and oh my friends, it gives a lovely light"? Koval is right. I've got to change my lifestyle and forget that pot of gold at the end of the rainbow because if I'm dead it doesn't mean a goddamn thing.

But it is not fading rainbows I think about now as I travel through my past. It is the warnings I had—ever more insistent, ever more ignored—that something was wrong with my heart.

Managua, Nicaragua

December 1962

My eyes snap open with a body jerk. A sharp short circuit between muscles, nerves, and brain. It comes with fatigue and pains in my chest, warning signs to ease back from the frantic pace. These past weeks there have been more of them than usual. I am older, tire more easily, and have been at the game too long. Ten years in a profession that averages 30 percent mortality during its career has got to be worse than front-line combat.

The alarm is set for 4:00 A.M., but some mental circuit breaker pops me into consciousness five minutes early. It never fails. Maybe the alarm isn't needed but with $700-a-day pilot pay riding on the outcome of such a gamble, I am afraid to test the theory.

I light a Marlboro, my first from three packs to be consumed during the day. A decade the Surgeon General's Report has been out and I'm still trying to convince myself that it's all nonsense. Others may kill themselves in crashes, develop cancer, have heart attacks, or succumb to senility and old age. Others, but not I. At thirty, I am one of the few immortals. Such conceit and foolishness.

Through open louvered-glass windows stars shine in that last brittle brilliance before dawn. The city is quiet. How can 300,000 people crammed into so small an area be so silent?

In other hotels, pensions, and apartments scattered about the city other pilots are getting up too. We are called the gringo invaders who come each year to spray the country's huge cotton acreage.

Nicaragua's crop is planted in August. During the last week of that month the rainy season begins, predictable as my alarm clock. It starts with thunderheads building in the afternoon. By early evening their seams explode with jagged tears of light-

16

ning. Buckets of water flail down. At midnight it is over until the next day. Stars come from behind a misty curtain and the night air is rich with smells of washed pavement, porous brick, and damp vegetation.

Later, during September and October, there are days when an overcast canopies the entire country. Rain pours intermittently from dawn to dark and on through the night. At such times the pilots sleep or gather in the bar of the Gran Hotel on Calle Roosevelt to swap lies, talk shop and women, or curse the weather.

They come from everywhere: the States, Mexico, Argentina, New Zealand, and a few from Canada. Itinerant crop dusters. The term is malapropos: liquid spray has replaced the chemical dust. Never mind; whether spray pilot or crop duster, the job is the same. Productive flying in its purest, most exciting form.

A workday is every day that weather permits. Fly out at dawn. Fly back after dark in the rain to Managua's Xolotlan Airport in the city's industrial suburb. Its single runway a lumpy square of mud and slippery grass on which untethered animals graze. The field is surrounded on three sides by a dilapidated assortment of barnboard and packing-case hangars with leaky rusting roofs of corrugated tin. Machine-gun towers manned by Somosa's National Guardsmen provide security—and defense of the family's dictatorship—around the airport's open perimeter.

Las Mercedes, the city's international airport, lies a few miles farther south along the road to Tippitappa. Agricultural aircraft are excluded. It is reserved for international airlines and Nicaragua's pathetic little Fuerza Aerea, the latter a mottled collection of World War II surplus machines donated by the U.S. State Department to thwart the communist threat in this "bastion of democracy," so the official wording goes on a framed scroll hanging in the Officers' Mess.

As in the adjacent Central American dictatorships, State Department munificence and dollar-aid programs relate to the size of the communist threat. Judging from the military hardware in Nicaragua, the country rates low in U.S. spending priorities. Somosa's controlled newspaper *El Dia* devotes entire columns to the communist menace in every edition, but if there are Communists walking the country's roads and byways they are invisible.

I catch the alarm on its first strident note and roll from bed for a lukewarm shower, climb into a clean flying suit, gulp a pint of grapefruit juice, and pack my flight bag. It holds a thermos of ice-cold juice, sandwiches, pistol, ammo clips, tinned tuna, emergency first-aid kit, and my well-thumbed Canadian passport.

Alfonso Cardenal is waiting for me curbside, leaning against the side of *E Pluribus Unum*, ready to take me to the airport. His bucking Hillman Minx is the product of many hours spent at local wrecking yards seeking parts to keep this source of his livelihood operational.

"*Hola, Commandante!*"

He wears buck teeth, one of them capped in gold and displayed like a trophy whenever he smiles. He smiles a great deal, for he is a happy man.

Each September when I arrive from Canada to begin the Nicaraguan spraying season Alfonso finds me within the first twenty-four hours. He is my *hombre*. In a foreign country every pilot needs an *hombre*, just as every pilot needs a good woman. With Alfonso all things are possible. He delivers me to a bright, clean apartment already equipped with telephone, brand-new refrigerator, and beaming black laundry maid from Bluefields on the Atlantic coast. All for me at an outrageous price. We argue. It takes a day or two before I am prepared to accept his lowered price and he mine.

He is much older than I, a flabby fifty with close-set small sly eyes and graying hair. His habit is foul-smelling cigars and the taxi reeks even when he isn't smoking. I have insisted that he never smoke them in my presence, so he chews at them until I leave his premises.

"Long or short day, *Commandante?*"

His Hillman huffs through stoplights on the Calle

Roosevelt. At this hour no one pays any attention to lights. On one corner a pair of carbine-toting Guardsmen loiter.

Alfonso asks this question every morning and always I reply, *"Quién sabe?"*

How can any spray pilot know the length of his day? But this isn't the reason for his asking. It's to test my mood. Some mornings I'm inclined to chat for the entire twenty minutes it takes to drive across the city. At these times I learn more about the Cardenal family than my own.

Blood relations, in-laws, mistresses, and frightful tales of incest and bestiality come spilling from Alfonso's cigar-stained lips. If but a quarter is true I'm amazed that Harvard or Princeton hasn't sent a fully equipped anthropological research team down to beat the bushes for satyrs or unicorns.

Never have I managed to trip him on these stories when, weeks or months later, I make him repeat an incident that has stuck in my mind. Either they are all true or Alfonso has an incredible ability for deceit.

This morning I wish silence, so there is no elaboration on my initial *quién sabe*. He respects my wish. I've found, as these seasons draw to a close in each country, less inclination to indulge in conversational trivia. There is a feeling of being one of the last guests at the party, when hosts have removed their shoes and look pointedly at their mantel clocks with dianoetic anticipation.

By Christmas only dispossessed foreigners will remain to finish patchwork spraying: small sections on enormous fields where cotton bolls still burst after the main harvest has been collected. Everybody else moves on to the next season, the next country. Except the Americans who, along with the Brits, go home because the attraction of white whiskers, yule log, holly, and mistletoe is too strong to resist. The rest fly to Peru where the season is just beginning.

I won't go this year. That magic of flying Andean passes in an unheated open cockpit has palled. Besides, roaring inflation has reduced the Peruvian *sol* to where it is nearly valueless and the farmers cannot pay in dollars.

Instead, I will go to Mexico City and stay at La Malinche, a sumptuous brothel in the elegant residential district near Chapultapec forest. Everything is provided for relaxation at a price. Every capital city has its La Malinche if one takes the trouble to look.

Near the airport's entrance Alfonso gives a young duty Guardsman a wave. First tin shack on the right is where I climb out. Alfonso waits. Other cars and taxis arrive. The pilots spill out, lighting cigarettes, nodding agreeably to one another as they troop into the control office to make out flight plans for their day's activities.

It is a formality, nothing more. If a man goes down in the jungle the only search to be mounted will come from the pilots themselves. Everyone knows where everyone else is working. I insert a fictitious license number on the form, write Boeing 707 for my aircraft type, and under destination print BULGARIA in neat block letters. The jokes on these forms are lost on the Guardsman collecting the flimsy carbon copies because we all know he can neither read nor write.

Guardsmen are picked for loyalty and obedience, not intelligence. Flat-faced Indians from the interior with swarthy features and watchful eyes, they wear faded gray denim, frayed web belts, plastic helmet liners, and new black boots polished to ebony perfection. Utterly ruthless and, when properly led, magnificent soldiers.

Unfortunately, their officers share little enthusiasm for anything but the good life. Most are political sycophants appointed, then annointed by the Somosa family to insure a perpetuity of mediocrity. Certainly this planned hierarchy must have exceeded the family's wildest expectations.

Even government jobs of nondescript importance carry the perk of rank and title: customs, immigration, law courts, departments of sanitation, highways, agriculture, and utilities. Somewhere near the top of these impecunious mobs of illiterate workers the uniformed ranking begins. A country truly run as a single family enterprise. This is its strength and principal weakness.

Innovation, criticism, and real political opposition are stifled in the name of a democracy's fear of communism. Reality is more obvious: a fascist dictatorship managing successfully to smother emotional nationalism for decades under U.S. sponsorship. In time, like Cuba, the governments of these State Department satrapies all will be overthrown: Panama, El Salvador, Guatemala, Honduras, and Nicaragua. It is as certain as the sunrise.

Alfonso takes me the last few hundred yards to our company hangar. On the rough ground *E Pluribus Unum* develops some alarming new groans.

"Look for me in the early afternoon," I tell him finally.

It's unfair to keep him waiting outside the airport gate in the hot sun with no idea of my return when he can be hustling passengers for short fares and generous tips downtown. Maybe he does have eleven kids, wife, and mistress to support in addition to all his strange in-laws. He gives a gold smile of relief and wishes me good luck aloft.

Dino Zaglaviras, my business partner, is screaming invective at Andres, our chief mechanic. Andres is on loan from the Nicaraguan Air Force. Why he puts up with Dino's abuse is still a mystery.

"What's going on?" I yell between them.

In the yellow light from the office doorway their complexions have taken on Oriental hues.

"*Idiota!*" Dino howls.

"I forgot to check the tank. We have no gasoline *señor*," Andres says apologetically.

"Impossible. Texaco filled it last night. I signed their delivery slip and locked the tank myself."

Dino stops yelling and looks at me blankly.

"Then we've been robbed! A thousand gallons! The fuckers got us again!"

He yanks out his .45 automatic and slides the mechanism. In his eyes I see murder. Our American pilots sitting on the bench outside the office smoking cigarettes stir uneasily. It is an act. Dino is all actor.

When I met him ten years ago on the Canadian forestry spray program his name was Constantine Zaglaviras and he couldn't speak enough English to order his supper. A Greek from Athens whose family were murdered in the troubles of 1947, Dino took his pilot training with the Greek Air Force in San Antonio, Texas, under the NATO program. That training is the only reason he is still alive because he's a terrible pilot with no natural feel for any aircraft. One day he will kill himself.

"Put the gun away, you nitwit, before it goes off."

"A thousand gallons, Tony!"

"Where's your night watchman?"

Eduardo was hired by Dino to prevent theft. I mistrusted the man from the first evening he turned up, bobbing obsequiously to everyone in sight. He has vanished together with the avgas, probably sold to one of our competitors, watchman to watchman. The truth will never be known.

Dino holsters his weapon, swearing to find Eduardo, recover the fuel, then blow off the man's head. Only the Americans seem impressed, not realizing that he switched into English for their benefit. Fortunately the aircraft fuel tanks are full.

"Let's go to work," I suggest to everyone.

Around the airport aircraft engines cough, choke, bark, and roar to life, splitting the silence of dawn. To the east, beyond the trees, a powder-pink light filters through the leaves.

"Phone Texaco for another load, Andres."

"Yes, señor."

He gives me a wink, then raises his eyes and hands in resignation at Dino striding away to his aircraft.

We went into business together in Honduras in the late 1950s. By then Dino had given up his Canadian citizenship for an absurd Honduranian passport, promoted himself to full colonel, married a local mestizo woman, and changed his name to Douglas Zagar. None of it made much difference to his flying or managerial abilities. He still burns up engines and tears up at least one airplane each year, all the while terrorizing our employees.

As a result of a political misunderstanding we were thrown out of Honduras two years ago and brought our six machines into Nicaragua. Dino has a house in Colonia Mantica and lives in the country year round. Four months is about all I can stand of the place.

Our aircraft are remodeled Stearman biplanes, surplus trainers from the last world war. Bigger engines, constant-speed propellers, and 200-U.S.-gallon spray tanks fitted into the front cockpit turn these wood- and fabric-covered machines into agricultural workhorses capable of lifting a ton of chemical spray. Pipes and nozzles hang awkwardly from the lower wings, while beneath the belly a small wind-driven pump keeps the juices flowing at pressure. It looks crude but it works.

They are a delight to fly, these antique biplanes. Quick response on controls, good maneuverability at their 110-mph working speed, and enough ruggedness to withstand the frightful punishment of rough graded airstrips, which, for the most part, are either too soft or too hard.

Today I'm taking one of the Americans for wingman. Tom Putnam is a bulbous-nosed old-time duster pilot from McAllen, Texas. He speaks not a word of Spanish despite a lifetime of living on the Mexican border. Yet he's an excellent pilot, easy on equipment, babying his engine, never allowing himself to be trapped into a situation beyond his ability. It is clear why he is still alive after twenty-five years in the game. I enjoy flying with him.

Andres swings my propeller. None of the aircraft has a starter or electrical system. When a plane crashes it is usually its electrical system that causes fire in the same way a car explodes rolling down an embankment. No battery, no fire unless the wing tank ruptures, spraying the hot cylinders. I try not to think about that.

Another mechanic pulls my wheel chocks and I signal Putnam to move. From all over the airfield machines taxi toward the take-off point, elbowing their way into line. They roar off, lifting like angry hornets, sometimes in pairs if a wingman happens to be ex-air force and knows the art of holding an echelon position.

With empty spray tanks, a Stearman breaks ground in under eight hundred feet. We climb through the city's morning haze of breakfast fires, their smoke flattened low against the inversion layer sitting just above the city. The air is cool. I lower my seat and look for Tom. He pulls in on my left, a red helmet and wide goggles watch my wingtip.

Together we turn out past the shoreline over Lake Managua, aiming for Momotombo's smoking crater at the north end of the lake. After 450 years of digesting the city's raw sewage this picturesque lake is dying. At one time, before the land contorted, it joined mighty Lake Nicaragua to the south and the open Pacific beyond. Now the only connection to this salt-water past are its fresh-water sharks.

In early morning when the lake is flat, it is great sport to glide down until the aircraft wheels brush the water, then ski its entire length trailing twin rooster-tails of spray. At flying speed the thick doughnut tires will not dig through the surface without considerable forward pressure on the control stick. No one knows how much forward pressure it takes to make an aircraft dig in and flip. Two pilots broke their necks trying last year. Nicaraguan greenhorns trying to ape the macho foreigners.

Momotombo is still an active volcano, one of a dozen in the country always rumbling with indigestion. Every spray pilot makes a point of flying the crater's walls of hot ash and cinders to smell the acrid sulphur fumes belching from the bowels of the earth. It is an awesome sight and feeling to be circling in the mouth of hell.

Dawn, like dark, comes quickly in the tropics. No gentle warming of light and shadows, no afterglow at sunset. A roller blind that goes up and down. I light another cigarette to greet the sun—no mean accomplishment in an open cockpit.

Putnam drops back a little and turns his head away to examine the volcano. Tight formation flying is hard work, requiring constant minute throttle adjustments. Fun to practice for a while but tiring unless somebody is paying money to watch the show.

Malpacillo, our destination, is Nicaragua's counterpart of

Dodge City and the old romantic West. Hunched between the new Pan American Highway on the east and the country's spiny coastal mountains, the town is a twentieth-century anachronism. Everybody packs weapons from pearl-handled six-shooters to three-foot, razor-sharp machetes. Even flourbag-panted urchins carry slingshots capable of imbedding marble-sized ball bearings into fence posts.

Most men in the community suffer from long-term effects of perpetual mortal combat. Some hobble on twisted limbs; others of nobler birth appear in public on the shoulders of armed retainers. Missing eyes, ears, noses, hands, and limbs are commonplace. Few females are in evidence. It was explained to me that they are the cause of most of the fights.

At the town's edge is a smooth, hard-packed airstrip, one of the country's best. Ground-support personnel are always superb and well organized; pilots are treated as visiting celebrities. Farmers pay their accounts in cash when the job is finished each day. It is understood that no resident of the town qualifies for credit consideration when he could be dead by dusk.

Despite these advantages, plus a 20 percent surcharge for coming to the town, most pilots give Malpacillo a wide berth. The local farmers hate Yankees and anyone who cannot speak Spanish is considered Yankee. America's successive military interventions between 1928 and 1932 still weigh heavily on their minds. U.S. Marines kept well clear of the place after a brief skirmish in which six of their number were captured, then roasted alive on barbecue poles. I have warned Tom Putnam to keep his mouth shut and let me do the talking.

Two years ago, when my Spanish was poor, I witnessed the short-fused passions of two brothers, sons of a farmer for whom I was working. They had been assigned the task of refueling my aircraft. Both kept slopping gas on the ground, me, the airplane, and each other. Finally, in exasperation, one hurled the contents of a five-gallon pail into the other's face, blinding him.

Howling, the younger brother raced off to wash his eyes. In minutes he returned, picked up his machete, and, with a single stroke, severed the other's left arm at the elbow. For a moment the older brother stood stunned, looking at his severed member, then the blood gushing from his stump. He drew out his revolver, an old British Army Webley, and shot his brother in the face, emptying the weapon before collapsing himself.

Their father told me the following week that he thought his older son had done the proper thing in the circumstances.

"After all, *señor*," he pointed out, "young Ramon started it, didn't he? If a man cannot finish what he started, he is not a man."

"And how goes it with your other son?"

"Oh, he died too. Bled to death before I returned to the airfield. You will join me for lunch?"

Minutes before reaching town, Putnam closes up. The locals appreciate a tight-formation fly-past at fifty feet, followed by a hammerhead turn on the break over the end of the runway, then a three-point landing in a puff of dust.

As we roar across the red-tiled roofs, Putnam's wingtip is close enough for me to reach out and touch. I raise my hand to signal the break, then yank back hard on the stick and zoom straight up into a power stall, cut the throttle, kick rudder, and drop like a stone vertically for the ground. At the last moment I pull back, flaring to brush the tires onto smooth yellow dirt. Tom is right behind me. We taxi to the end and park.

"Hola, qué tal?"

The farm administrator is a short, bandy-legged block of granite with the crumpled face of a pugilist. His hands are wide slabs, thick and square. He crushes me with an affectionate *abrazo*. We're old friends. I introduce Tom. They squeeze fingers long and hard until the veins start out on their foreheads. The American gives up first and Bakoda laughs, smashing him on the back. Throughout, Putnam keeps his lips compressed.

"This fat one, does he speak Spanish?" Bakoda roars.

"Not a goddamn word!" I yell over the sounds of our idling motors. "But he's a number-one *piloto*, Don Raoul."

The ground crew lift our loading pumps and hoses from the aircraft baggage compartments and set them up next to their mixing barrels. Drums of parathion, endrin, toxaphene, DDT, and other lethal chemical concoctions lie scattered about the ground, each container marked as to ownership. They have been trucked in at great cost from the mixing plant at Managua.

Chemical is mixed with water from an overhead wooden tower atop which is affixed a tattered Shell Oil windsock.

"Today we use parathion," the administrator announces, watching carefully that his men mix no more than the exact amount of chemical into each of the open barrels.

Every week chemicals are varied to prevent insects from developing mutants resistant to the poisons. Such variations help, but once nature's delicate balance has been tilted in favor of man, nothing is constant or certain. Incredibly, boll weevils have developed resistance to parathion.

Invented by the Germans prior to World War II as a nerve gas, the chemical attacks the central nervous system, causing paralysis in animals and insects. Two drops of liquid concentrate on the back of a dog's neck is sufficient to bring the animal into agonizing convulsions and death within five minutes. I have witnessed this frightful demonstration performed by two Bayer Chemical representatives at an agricultural convention in Mexico.

Its fumes are unmistakable, sickeningly sweet. I stand well back from the loaders and mixing drums. No one has told them that *veneno* can kill humans with the same facility as insects.

They wear leaky rubber gloves when handling the mixing paddle and loading hose, oblivious to splashes on their clothing or naked upper bodies. In another week they'll become nauseated, begin to vomit, lose their sense of balance, smell, and coordination. Bakoda will dismiss them and hire replacements. Their job is much sought after because it pays so well: five U.S. dollars a day.

In the dirt Bakoda uses a pointed stick to explain which fields are to be done. I translate for Putnam. They are lovely, long rectangular fields all within three miles of our airstrip. We should average five loads an hour without difficulty.

"Remember, there are wires on this one—near the end," he cautions.

Two pilots killed themselves at the field this year. But if one is very careful and drags the aircraft's wheels through the cotton foliage, there is just enough room to slip beneath these high-tension lines.

Wires are always difficult to negotiate and, through some trick of optics, invariably appear higher above the ground than they are. The Nicaraguan pilots flew too high or forgot they were there. Putnam will not forget.

"Have you flown under them?" he asks.

"Many times."

Satisfied, he nods and goes to his aircraft. I climb into mine, tighten the Sutton shoulder harness, and clamp my respirator over my mouth and nose. The sweetness of parathion changes to sweat and rubber. Twin charcoal filters keep out most of the fumes.

At a few minutes past six I cram on full power for my first load of the day. The plane moves sluggishly, slowly gathering speed. Behind me the loading crew scurry from the dust cloud blasting back to envelop them. Putnam taxis to position, waiting until I'm airborne.

Gradually the tail lifts clear, a few hundred feet more and my Stearman rises leadenly from the narrow strip. At fifty feet I level off and throttle back to cruising power. Through my swirling yellow dust Putnam begins his roll. Now the loading area is invisible in a cauldron of boiling grit.

At the cotton field flagmen have heard my take-off roar and trotted out to their signaling positions. The men are spaced four to a mile in a straight line twenty-five feet out from the fence. Each carries a long bamboo pole with a white flag attached to its tip. They are the compass by which pilots can fly in straight lines.

After each pass the flagmen move over fifty feet and begin waving location for the next swath. They wear no protective clothing, no respirators, no shoes. Lord knows how many of them I have helped to kill.

My aircraft's nose is aligned with the row of waving flags. I tilt forward, sliding down near crop level. As I cross the fence line and slam the spray handle, opening the main valve, chemical erupts from sixty wing nozzles, blending into twin whorls of rainbow behind the aircraft to go churning through the foliage.

The air is cool and calm, heavy air with lots of wing support, a pleasure to fly. Mid-December is the end of the rainy season for the Central Americas. Now the windy season commences. By 9:00 A.M. I'll be riding a bucking quarterhorse in thirty-five-mph gusts, trying to hold my wings level; but for the moment I'm enjoying this ride on a smooth, docile brood mare.

My wheels flick through the plant tops, tearing out leaves and branches. Farmers like to see vegetation stuck in an aircraft's undercarriage: they believe that a good professional jobs requires flying at zero altitude. Nonsense, of course, since six feet above the crop is ideal, but none will believe that. Since they're paying to have the job done their way, I deliver what is expected of me and keep my opinions to myself.

At the end of the run I snap off the spray and hurtle into a tight climbing turn. On top, I let the nose fall, aligning with the flagman who has raced to his next position because Putnam's aircraft is right behind. As I drop back to the field, Tom is pulling up—higher than my turn to avoid turbulence from my slipstream—his gushing spray snapped off over the low fence at the exact moment mine starts again.

It is exhilarating work with the added pleasure of knowing that conditions are ideal for the best possible job. After my first load, when Bakoda has seen the tattered leaves and twigs clinging in my wheels, I'll creep up to proper height and stay there until the winds begin blowing. After that it's by guess and by God.

Eight minutes in the air. Four minutes on the ground loading. The morning passes. The wind puffs up, changing skies from limpid blue to dirty bronze under a scorching sun. Dust devils dance merrily about the landscape, lethal little monsters capable of twisting an aircraft into the ground. My face burns, lips crack, sweat dries to powder streaks, and my mouth fills with grinding flecks of lava ash. At midmorning I pause between loads to drink from my thermos.

Suddenly a pain hauls my breath away. A vise inside my chest begins tightening the last ounce of air from my lungs. The pain is unbelievable. For an instant I think I've been shot, but there is no sign of blood, only its feeling pounding in my brain. Gasping, I sink to the ground seeking escape.

Bakoda rushes up . His lips move, yet I can hear nothing but the roaring in my ears. He pushes me flat on the ground, loosens my helmet chin straps, then moistens my lips with what remains of the juice.

Very slowly the pain passes. My lungs find oxygen and the vise begins unwinding. Then there is no more pain, only weakness and a little fear.

"Are you still with me, my friend?" he asks anxiously.

"Yes, Don Raoul, alive and well." I even manage a smile.

"That cold juice. You drink too fast. Small sips are best in this heat."

I agree. But we are both wrong.

The antiseptic walls of Dr. Eduardo Rivas Gabeldon's office waiting room are festooned with framed proof of his vast erudition and qualifications. There is one from the Mayo Clinic where he interned. The Mayo Clinic! Let's hear it for Minneapolis. Graduate studies at Johns Hopkins and Walter Reed hospitals. A swift genuflect to Washington, D.C. If he's so goddamn good, why is he here in Managua?

Dr. Eduardo Rivas Gabeldon's pneumatic nurse gives me a polite "hsssst." The doctor will see me now.

"Your tests are back and everything is negative."

"Negative?"

He looks pleased. I can never adjust to the medical profession's use of the word "negative." To me it conjures up hideous ramifications, whereas "positive" implies good things. In medicine the reverse is true.

"There is nothing to report—blood, lungs, heart, and urine are all normal. You are in splendid condition. I envy you, *señor.*"

Dr. Gabeldon is a squat man with thinning black hair, round, bowling-ball features, and oddly bloodshot eyes filled with flecks of dark pigmentation. His stubby brown fingers belong to a stonemason, coarse and callused. We're about the same age.

"Then what caused my chest pain?"

He lights an imported menthol cigarette after offering me one. I can't stomach their flavor. I light up one of my own brand.

"Many things. Not eating enough, too little sleep, too many of these things"—he waves his filter tip above the desk— "working too hard. Where are you going for Holy Week?"

In the Latin Americas Christmas is celebrated as Holy Week.

"To Mexico City for a holiday."

"Excellent idea. Rest and relaxation for two weeks. You'll notice the difference immediately. You can pay my nurse on your way out."

Maybe he's right after all. Maybe that's all I need. Somewhere I remember reading that 90 percent of all our ailments are imaginary, psychosomatic. Our pains are quite real but caused by our minds, not our bodies.

Dino has arranged invitations for us to attend the annual party at the Officers' Club, a privilege regarded by the envious as comparable to being called to the bar or on the Queen's Honors List. The club is a pretentious piece of old Spanish architecture situated at the bottom of the grassy hill below the Presidential Palace. In Managua, no one can live in more rarefied air than the Somosas. Their palace is the highest point overlooking the city.

Although the president doesn't appear during the dreary formal affair his younger brother, "Tachito," is there to accept homage on his behalf. Recently the younger Somosa had his military title raised from colonel to general because there were too many colonels in the country already. For a Somosa, anything is possible.

He is a dark porcine man with shifty eyes hidden permanently behind tinted glasses. Wherever he moves, bodyguards and mistresses vie for position. His English is perfect, his morals Byzantine. Dino introduces me as a junior partner in our local enterprise.

"Well, I couldn't say we are fifty-fifty. After all, he thinks I'm a colonel and you're just a civilian," he says after we've been pushed down the receiving line to the bar.

"Dino, I don't think he thinks about you at all or ever will."

I drink too much during the evening and make owl eyes at some of Somosa's mistresses or party girls—or whatever they are. He sees the play and brings the girl to my sofa, a fat smile splitting his features. I stand; after all, he's the host.

"You like this one?"

"I like them all, general."

He introduces me to the girl. Her name is Sandra; she has red hair and comes from Fort Lauderdale. What the hell is she doing down here with this slob?

"I give her to you for the night," he says in a moment of magnanimity, pushing the poor girl against me and upsetting my drink over the front of her dress.

"What's the matter, general, can't get it up tonight?"

He snaps his fingers. Two bodyguards imprison my arms, then hustle me through the crowds and out the front door to a police car. After a professional beating in the city's jail I'm pushed into a crowded room where I fight my way across sleeping bodies to reach the single barred window for some fresh air.

There is no chest pain to assess because I hurt all over. My nose is broken and the rubber truncheon they used must have cracked some ribs, every breath aches. Just the same, it was worth it to see the expression on that fat face. Someday when I don't hurt so much maybe I can laugh about it.

Outside the narrow window a billion stars light up the cosmos. In a week it will be Christmas. Peace on earth, good will toward men!

Kingston, Canada

My blood enzymes have confirmed a moderate heart attack. A nebulous term. Dr. Koval explains: "Your enzyme count was between five and six hundred. A serious heart attack would be in the fifteen-hundred-to-two-thousand range. Critical at three thousand. You're on the low end of the scale, so you've got that much to be thankful for."

It makes things so much easier to accept when terms can be explained in relation to fixed guideposts. If three thousand is critical, then one hundred would be mild. I understand.

"You will make a full recovery and be able to go back to what you were doing without having to worry about curtailing physical activities. In fact, you might want to increase your physical activity on a gradual basis. Exercise is the very best thing after a heart attack. Walking in particular."

I am delighted with this news. Over the past few days my outlook has improved relative to the surroundings. No longer do I feel like a patient but more like an interloper occupying bed space when others more deserving could be using it to better advantage. The future is bright with optimism. Everything now is possible. I shall live, grow sleek and strong, maintain daily exercise regimen and strict diet, and close my mind to all intrusions that might lead to tension.

My heart rate is down to an impossible forty-six beats a minute, blood pressure barely rippling my arteries at a sedate 100 over 70. I'm anxious to be out of bed and started on my new program. Once they move me from intensive care, the children can come and visit. I have missed them.

"I'm putting you on Anturan—a precaution."

"Wonderful. What's Anturan?"

I've seen the magic of Inderal at work, but the Mighty

33

Andrew Koval apparently has a Gladstone stuffed with potions. A precaution against what? Dare I volunteer ignorance by asking?

"Among other things, it's an anticoagulant. Keeps your blood thin to prevent clotting."

Is this good or bad, I wonder? If I cut my hand on a kitchen knife or split open my head, am I doomed to a slow hemophilic demise? He laughs at these concerns.

"You've nothing to worry about. Twenty milligrams twice daily is all you'll be getting."

Such an infintesimal amount. Still, I worry. Perhaps I'm allergic to Anturan. Maybe my joints will swell, as happens to me with penicillin. I've read horror stories in *Reader's Digest* and *The National Inquirer* of case histories where gullible patients accepted "safe" drugs on prescription only to wind up basket cases, or chasing butterflies without a net. Shouldn't these allergy possibilities be checked in advance?

Why wouldn't forty milligrams be better than twenty? Too much? Is ten milligrams ineffective? How much is a goddamn milligram anyway and why twenty instead of nineteen or twenty-three? I've noticed all hospital dosages are administered in multiples of five or ten. Is this due to medical inability to work with numbers not divisible by five or a dark conspiracy with the drug companies?

"But didn't you tell me a few days ago this is what the Heparin shots into my stomach were supposed to prevent?"

"Heparin stops blood clots forming in your stomach where blood pools as you lie horizontal over long periods. But now that you're sitting up and able to move about there's no need for Heparin. The Anturan can take over."

"Good."

I dislike having long needles smacked into my tummy twice a day. Not that there is more than momentary discomfort; it's the idea of the assault that annoys.

"Not too much activity today, mind. Sit up in bed, sit in a chair. Short walks to the bathroom. No walking the halls just yet."

I mumble gratitude. They leave me with their wise smiles. All except the head nurse, a delightfully compassionate woman who makes me feel as if I'm approaching my eighth birthday at the speed of light and simply won't be ready for the added responsibilities.

"I'm so happy for you."

And I feel that she means it.

"Now then, soon as we've finished rounds I'll see what we've got ready, and move you down the hall. There's a phone in each room, so you can call your wife."

My blanketed foot receives a maternal pat on her way out. She is one of the reasons sick people get better.

Such elation! Graduation from intensive care. I sit up and dangle my bare feet over the edge of the chrome railings. On my night table I find a pencil and paper and set to work calculating the differential between ounces and Dr. Koval's milligrams.

I don't need to know but it proves that the analytical portion of my brain still works. After several minutes and four mutilated Kleenex tissues, it appears that a single milligram equals .02835 of an ounce—which doesn't really mean a hell of a lot or put me any further ahead. Still, if anybody should ask . . .

Hesitantly I swivel my neck, hearing it crack in contentment. Next my shoulders get a short rolling workout, finishing off with a delicious stretch. There's no pain anywhere. A slight backache from lying for three days on the hard hospital bed, but beyond this not the slightest feeling of anything amiss, internally or externally.

I have a ridiculous urge—quickly suppressed—to jump off the bed and go skipping along the corridor kicking my heels together. This heady wine of giddiness, relief, happiness, and well-being are all tamped into the barrel of my emotions, awaiting a flick of flintlock to explode. What heart attack?

We are all creatures imprisoned by our emotions and beliefs. To believe I am better is to be better. Dr. Koval's reassurances confirm my survival. The man is infallible. This is what I believe.

One of the older nurses tells a story of an elderly patient

who arrived on the floor after a massive heart attack. Blood enzyme count total: six thousand. An impossibility. The lab rechecked their findings. Same results. The man's heart function turned out to be nearly 90 percent impaired. Yet he lived. She had seen him recently, two years after his attack. His only complaint was that the winter walk from his farmhouse to the end of his laneway to pick up the morning mail left him a little breathless. He lived a quarter-mile from the road. How adaptable the human body and spirit.

A shrill warning alarm sounds outside at the desk monitors. In seconds the nurses are scrambling. Loud-speaker calls echo along the corridors asking doctors to report immediately to Cardiac Care, followed by a code number. From my open door I can see them rushing into the old woman's room next to mine. They bring machines, pumps, long needles atop enormous syringes filled with innocuous fluids, all of it at the run.

Sounds of thumping, groans, determined urgings, shoulder through the walls. In the corridor outside intensive care, ambulatory patients pause and peer with quizzical faces at the drama in progress. Nurses shoo them on their way but they leave reluctantly, their eyes locked on the fishbowl and the old woman's fight. It is the same solemn stare of uncertainty awarded strangers by every two-year-old who ever manned a stroller in a busy department store or crowded supermarket. Who are you out there above me and why do I fear you so much? When first do we learn the reality of death?

I was seven when my grandfather died in Nova Scotia's Annapolis Valley. On the East Coast a burying is much the same as a new birth or a ship's launching. Clarion calls ring out across the land for family to assemble—no mean task because they have been multiplying since 1761 when three brothers sold their Connecticut farms and moved north for free vacant lands left by the Acadia Expulsion.

My grandfather, a doctor and distinguished military man with heavy mustache, lay boxed on velvet in the front parlor. On the night before his funeral I crept from my room, down squeaky stairs, to examine him. He looked the same as I remembered, perhaps a bit paler. My, how odd. I'd expected death to look like squashed cats along the highway, soggy feathered birds, or car-struck dogs with broken limbs at impossible angles. In fact my grandfather appeared far from dead. Possibly sleeping?

Leaning against the coffin, I whispered hello. No reply. I leaned closer and whispered louder. Gray hairs sprouted from his ears, stubble from his chin. Hesitantly I touched his face. Ice cold and solid like stale rubber. I fled the room back up to bed and clutched the covers around my head. For the first time I had touched death.

After a few minutes, sounds and struggles cease from the old woman's room. Someone switches off the monitor alarm. In twos and threes staff members begin leaving, tight in earnest conversation. With great care and as little physical effort as possible, I slide my legs back on the bed and under the sheet. That urge to cavort the corridor has gone.

My nurse returns and pulls the night curtain across the glass wall and doorway.

"Did she die?"

"She was old and very sick."

"Aren't we all."

The curtain is to prevent the living from watching departure of the dead to the basement morgue. A thoughtful attempt to spare patients' feelings. But there's a gap where my curtain doesn't quite meet the wall. Soon after, I see a narrow gurney arrive, then, minutes later, leave. A black rubberized sheet has been fitted neatly over the entire package, end posts, sides, and corpse. Only barest outlines pressing the sheet from below reveal its cargo.

For a while voices outside my door are muted. Corridor perambulators cease their shufflings. Even the chain smokers in the visiting lounge near the elevators are quiet, their phlegmy coughs suppressed.

Gradually the floor's tempo resumes its normal pace. Brief laughter floats, is stifled quickly, then floats again. A telephone rings at the desk outside. My curtains are opened. Ted DeJager stands in the doorway.

Dr. DeJager is my G.P. This is his first visit. A stocky, moon-faced man, he is one of the medical benefits visited upon prisoners by the penal system.

On the day I entered hospital he wrote me a letter, collected by Helen, adjudging my chest pains to be a "small hiatus hernia but very definite and clear aerophagia," concluding with the suggestion that he arrange for me to visit a "Gastroenterologist who will confirm this diagnosis and will deal with the rest accordingly thereafter." *Quod Erat Demonstratum.*

"How are you feeling?"

What he means to ask is if I intend to sue.

"Okay now."

I *should* sue him when I get out of here. Hire a fancy percentage lawyer with a resonant ring to his voice for jury addresses and turn him loose. In the United States I could retire on the outcome. But medical testimony is hard to find because members of the profession join antlers in a perfect circle prepared to repel every assault against an errant brother, irrespective of circumstance.

"I've been out of touch a couple days. I just heard what happened."

He studies my clipboard for errors, leafing through the documentation contradicting his written opinion.

"Very hard to identify angina pectoris unless an ECG can be done when it's happening to you. Y'know, it's too bad you didn't have an attack while I had you in my office."

"Inconsiderate," I agree. "But tell me, aren't nitroglycerin tablets supposed to relieve angina pains?"

"Quite correct."

"Then why in hell didn't you try nitroglycerin to see what would happen? Surely, after all the X-rays, barium swallows, gallons of antacid, a light should have dawned on other possibilities?"

At one juncture he'd decided my problem was stomach ulcers or, failing that, a ruptured esophagus. He arranged an appointment with a radiologist to confirm his assessment. I stood before a giant fluoroscope and downed vile-tasting white chalk in water on an empty stomach while the radiologist scanned my innards—a procedure known in the trade as a "barium swallow." The chalky mixture produces vivid X-ray illumination of the digestive tract for sufficient time to be studied on the spot or photographed for later evaluation.

A waste of time in my case because both stomach and esophagus were without blemish. More REMs from my body's storehouse burned up to no purpose.

Intent on my file, DeJager ignores all questions. He studies each page carefully, reading everything, occasionally nodding.

"I think I'm going to be able to help you, Tony."

It takes a heart attack to get on a first-name basis with Dr. DeJager.

"I have some influence in the right places," he says modestly. "First of all, we have to get you out of here."

"I'm being moved today, down the hall."

"Well, there you are then!" he exclaims, prepared to take full credit for the decision.

On cue, two nurses arrive to collect my paraphernalia, disconnect me from the monitor, pull up the side bars, and wheel me out. He stops short of trailing my bed and escorting me down the hall but shouts an encouraging promise to return when he isn't so busy.

My new room is across the corridor from the nurses' lounge. Decor is early Holiday Inn with stainless-steel and chrome overtones. Everything is sparkling clean and tidy. I have a roommate. Mr. Sung. A neat, diminutive Chinese gentleman who, upon being introduced by the nurses as they roll me past his bed and next to the window, sits up with a lovely smile and bows. Our beds are separated by a night stand. And there is a telephone. Behind the stand, floor-length curtains suspended from overhead tracks can be drawn to encircle either bed for privacy.

I'm given a tiny portable transmitter in a cloth bag to hang around my neck. Its radio signals are picked up by the desk monitors back at intensive care, recording my heart's activities wherever I may wander on the floor. Not too far today, but I intend to explore the premises as quickly as I'm able and permitted. The nurses leave. I sit reveling in new-found freedom.

Mr. Sung smiles. "You heart?"

His voice has that soft musical hiss unique to every Oriental.

"I heart," I agree.

Satisfied, he nods. "I heart too." And gives his transmitter a gentle tap, sighs, then lies back to stare at the ceiling.

I have no idea of his age. Anywhere from fifty to eighty. There is an ageless quality to his clear eyes and smooth skin. Even his short-cropped hair, pointing every which way, looks vigorous.

"You here long time?"

Why do Occidentals lapse into a form of pidgin English whenever we address elderly Orientals? Every word must be enunciated carefully as though talking to a four-year-old. What is it about their speech patterns that triggers our minds into producing such condescending drivel?

"Two week."

"Ah, then you'll be leaving soon."

My syntax is readjusted with difficulty.

"Dr. Milligan say pretty soon. You know Dr. Milligan?"

"No, I don't."

"Good doctor!"

He subscribes to Mighty Milligan, I the all-powerful Koval. We're both disciples of their coronary cause; different branches of the same religion like Methodists and Presbyterians espousing Calvinist doctrines.

I leave him to his thoughts. Orientals, I've discovered, have an abhorrence to instant familiarity.

Helen answers my phone call, delighted to hear that I've been sprung from close surveillance. For her it means confirmation of my improved condition. She promises to drop by after four o'clock when the children get home from school, bringing pajamas, dressing gown, electric razor, and some books.

While I'm on the phone a fat, jolly nurse with red hair and

wearing a student badge on her uniform enters the room towing
a portable scale with one hand, carrying a sphygmomanometer
and stethoscope in the other. She tilts the scales upright, then
stands smiling until I'm off the phone.

"I need your weight."

"It's yours for the asking."

"And your blood pressure and temperature."

"Take whatever you need. I am your captive. But please,
leave my shirty alone."

Giggling, she leads me to the scales.

Oddly, I'm a little lightheaded. The result of what? A weak
heart no longer capable of pumping blood to my brain in an
upright position or merely a normal over-all malaise from being
in bed these past days?

The scales balance at eighty-six kilograms, which sounds
wonderful but means nothing until it's been converted by the
jolly nurse's plastic card conversion tables into 189.59 pounds.
Since my heart attack I've lost three pounds.

She takes my temperature next. Normal. Finally, the
sphygmomanometer sleeve over my bicep to check diastolic and
systolic blood pressures, her stethoscope pressing against my
forearm.

Every year since leaving the air force in 1952 I have taken
medical examinations to maintain my commercial pilot's
license. When I finally reached the exalted airline transport
rating these medicals came every six months. A blood pressure
test was always part of the $25 package. It seemed such a gyp. A
perfectly healthy man forced to pay, by government decree,
some charlatan so much for doing so little. And not even tax
deductible at that.

"Very good, one hundred and twenty-three over seventy."
A few years later it became, "one hundred and thirty-five over
eighty. What more can you ask?" Finally, there came that dark
afternoon in Van Nuys, California, with a Santa Ana blowing
testily from the desert, I ran into a garrulous Federal Aviation
Administration appointee who clucked unhappily, "Tut, tut, one
hundred and forty over ninety-five. Right on the borderline, you

know? Going to have to learn to ease off on those throttles, try and relax, let it all hang out, live a little."

Only in California . . .

Unimpressed, I agreed always with whatever the examining physician advised—just so long as he signed my license renewal form. Systolic and diastolic pressures were buzz words that could be good or evil depending upon the doctor. Now I discover the truth from a student nurse with red hair, the truth that no doctor took the time or trouble to explain in layman terms.

Two arterial pressures are measured by the sphygmomanometer; systolic, produced when the heart is working, and diastolic, that pressure between beats when the heart is at rest. It is during this latter, diastolic, pause that the heart fills with blood preparatory to the systole, meaning simply the squeezing or contraction cycle of the heartbeat when fresh blood is expelled into the arteries.

Normal systolic pressure can be anything from 110 to 160, depending on age and circumstance, but it is the diastolic pressure, that bears watching carefully. Readings from 70 to 90 may be considered normal. Beyond 90 and over 100 can be indications of hypertension, narrowing arterial passages, or loss of pliability of the arteries themselves due to spasm or plaque formation. High systolic readings indicate a back pressure on the heart while it is in the diastole or blood-filling sequence. So simple when it is explained by a novice.

"Now you know." She giggles, then asks the Big Question.

I hang my head contritely. No, I have not had a bowel movement this morning but I'll try. Honest, I really will. The Little Engine That Could: I think I can—I think I can—I think I can.

Then a buxom dietitian with a fascinating gold pencil dangling from a tiny retractable chain pops in to deliver tomorrow's menu, together with detailed instructions on how to mark X next to my selections.

"Not checkmarks! Checkmarks won't do. We get lots of checkmarks but in the kitchen they don't mean a thing. We've got to have big clear X's!"

I play the duck, forcing her to haul the chain to its full length while she assists my confused efforts. Mr. Sung's wise eyes twinkle as he listens. In the end she realizes that I've been pulling her leg—and her chain—and walks out on me, not unhappily. After all, how often does she get to operate that chain?

The food selection is nourishing, if unimaginative. It has been stamped REGULAR DIET. No restrictions on salt, ice cream, whole milk, bread, animal fats, meats, or any of those evils mentioned by Dr. Koval during his litany on the root causes of heart attacks in a modern world. Surely someone has made a mistake. But no, the nurse assures me that I have no dietary restrictions. Strange.

Is remedial action taken now of no use? By readjusting eating habits and correcting basic dietary errors can I not slow the erosion to my system, perhaps even reverse its trend? There's a puzzling inconsistency here that I must discuss with Dr. Koval.

I take up the menu card and place broad muscular X's next to anything offering a blank space between two brackets. The results tomorrow should provide doggie bags for the children to take home after visiting hours.

Exhausted from this effort, I lie back against the pillows and contemplate Sir John's house, this time from a slightly different angle. So good to be alive and getting better.

A hospital is a country in miniature, every floor a city with its own mayor, aldermen, and council—all on eight- or twelve-hour shifts. Small, quaint villages laze in quiet backwaters off the central corridors, their names diverse and mysterious: "Telemetry," "Audiology," "Neurology," and "Nurses Only."

On the green-tiled parklands located at the end of each floor, tourists picnic while children play. Color television, comfortable chairs, sofas, plastic-skinned plants of impossible height, and monochrome pictures of startled fauna, all designed with an eye to the comfort of those who must sit and wait.

When my umbilical wires were disconnected and I left the womb of intensive care to flex my flabby muscles in the real world of the fourth floor, I became fair game for all the street hawkers who plied the corridors.

First, a breathlessly pretty girl—braless under a nipple-tight black sweater—and to all intents and purposes pantyless under a pair of designer jeans—rolls into the room with a cart of bedside TV sets. Her company, she explains, has the franchise to provide television service within the hospital. There is no alternative: either I rent from her or do without—much the same as a government road-paving contract.

"But I have a lovely nine-inch Sony color in my bedroom at home, complete with two yards of earplug wire. I'll ask my wife to bring it in this afternoon."

Her ruby lips tighten menacingly.

"Not allowed. My company has the franchise."

I study her list of rental fees, by the day or week, coming to the conclusion that by the fourth week I will have bought the set from her company and maybe a new pair of designer jeans for the girl, including bra. With thanks for her visit I decline the offer.

"Suit yourself, but it can get pretty dull lying around in here all day with nothing to do."

"I can catch up on my reading."

"You mean like books?"

She looks scornful, glances at Mr. Sung for the barest instant, then jounces out.

Short walks, the doctor said. So I spread my wings and teeter cautiously across the floor, around the end of Mr. Sung's bed, then on to the distant bright lights of the bathroom. It is deceptive. Distances are immense. At the door I look back in triumph at my roommate. He smiles, not inscrutably either.

Hospital bathrooms are designed to accommodate ambulatory patients with any or all diseases and physical limitations known to man. A blind, one-legged diabetic suffering angina pectoris and piles would have no difficulty negotiating the various levels of handholds, chest bars, and support racks protruding from the walls at strategic contact points. Sink and taps are without sharp corners or skull-splitting protrusions, toilet elongated with catch basin for feces reclamation, toilet paper the consistency of eider down, even the illuminated mirror has been silvered in muted tone to make loose flesh and dark-circled eyes appear tricks of shadow. In a rack behind the basin, urinary "spotting" test bottles are set out together with a detailed color chart for diabetic patients to check their emission shading.

Very slowly I lather soap onto a washcloth, then rub the clag from my bristled face. It is exhausting work. Bedside basin washes by nurses are no trade-off for the ability to bend over a sink and slather my face and neck with hot soapy water. Already I feel better. Chest, armpits, tummy, and groin are treated in similar fashion. Water sloshes the floor into a drain hole. My head itches, so I shampoo with regular soap. I'd prefer to finish with a shave followed by the cool, sweet sting of lotion. Instead, because my bowels are rumbling mightily, I wind up sitting on the can.

At eye level from the toilet seat there is a bright red emergency button with short ring chain. My panic button. Directions are printed in bold white lettering. I feel no panic, only tiredness.

It takes several minutes to recover my breath before attempting the long return journey to bed. I stagger off, sweat beads swelling on lips and brows. There is a frightful hammering under my rib cage. Not rapid staccato; more the heavy methodical swing of a galley master's drumbeat to his rowers.

I know something is wrong. I've overtaxed my healing heart. How could I have been so stupid? Fortunately there is comfort in knowing that everything will show on the desk monitor and nurses will come running to my rescue, once again saving my miserable life. With Herculean effort I slide onto the bed and lie waiting for them to appear.

Minutes pass and a pale-faced, beaky woman with narrow, sloping shoulders and darting, timid eyes stands hesitantly in the doorway. She's dressed in a light purple habit with plastic name tag affixed to one lapel. Too far away to read.

"I'm with the Chaplain's Office," she whispers.

Ye gods. They've seen my monitor and decided on sending this devout creature to prepare me for the worst. Pressure builds in my chest, not angina and no pain. A lightheadedness brought on by a resolve to meet disaster with fixed smile, no matter what the emotional effort?

She steps sparrowlike toward my bed, hands aflutter, eyes brimming in consternation. I pale at her approach. Out floats a hand to hang suspended like a crumpled wing, waiting to be clasped. The fingers are ice, nails bitten to their quick. I feel myself sinking, sucked into a dark, swirling tunnel, my breath comes in gasps. Clutching her claw for succor, I manage to squeeze out a tremulous "Thank you for coming."

"Is there anything I can do? Pray for you?" It is obvious that she knows I am beyond help or hope. "Are you a Christian?"

"Oh yes." And I hope not beyond redemption.

I hate to disappoint this ministering angel. Besides, "freebee" prayers are all the rage and if I'm going anyway, why not have somebody outside the immediate family say a few words to smooth my passage? In silence we cling to each other. Suddenly the duty nurse confronts me, wresting me from the purple lady's hold.

"You're not transmitting."

"I'm not?"

She yanks up my shirty and sure enough one of the small alligator clips has twisted loose from the metal contact point taped to my chest. It must have pulled free during my ablutions. She snaps it into position. Then testily as she departs: "Do try and be more careful."

They really do watch those monitors and I'm not suffering a relapse. That hammering feeling has gone, along with my purple lady. Life will go on after all.

A human mind can play idiotic tricks, magnifying the slightest irregularity out of all proportion to its importance. Each fantasy builds upon the previous one until, like an inverted pyramid balancing on the head of a pin, the whole insanity comes crashing down to turn the poor hallucinator permanently hypochondriacal or, worse, insane.

During his fourth year at medical school a doctor told me of a fellow student he knew who managed to convince himself he had a leaky mitral valve. The mitral valve separates the left and right chambers of the heart. He claimed to be able to hear it distinctly with his stethoscope. Convinced finally that everybody else was lying to him about his condition, he took to bed— permanently. Within three years he was dead, killed by his own imagination.

My next visitor is a paper boy who deals in cash. I give my word to pay him the next day when I'll have funds.

"How do I know you're going to be here tomorrow?"

Don't I realize this is the cardiac ward? Smart kid. What difference will the newspaper make anyway? My world is here with Mr. Sung. Strife beyond these walls must remain the concern of others, for I am powerless to affect the course of history now—not altogether an unpleasant feeling.

A two-hour period after lunch is ordained to be rest time. Window curtains are drawn, shutting out the blowing snow that clicks on the glass in frenzied gusts. Mr. Sung's eyes close and within moments he has glided into deep slumber. Legs and arms perfectly straight, chest out, stomach in, he snores quietly at attention.

Home is the sailor home from the sea,
And the hunter home from the hill.

Montreal, Canada

15 February 1972

Barney Flieger is a big man with a canyon voice and a bow tie. His hair is gray and curly. A neatly trimmed and serviceable mustache adorns his lip while his eyes are bright with perpetual skepticism.

I had taken the night train from Toronto to meet him today for lunch. There is a submission in my briefcase for both federal and provincial governments, something that will revolutionize aircraft-spraying methods around the world. To see it off to a smooth start I need Barney's blessing and a million-dollar contract to prove its worth. I intend to get both in Montreal. Barney Flieger is Mr. Forestry Aviation Spraying of Canada, perhaps the world. And he likes me.

Our first meeting came at the university in New Brunswick where he held a professorship in the Forestry Department while I, a goggle-eyed teenager, flirted with law and socialism between campus romances. In those days he wore spiffy Spike Jones suits, eye-popping bow ties, and kept his curly hair well groomed with Wildroot Cream Oil, Charlie.

There were rumors—never challenged or proved—that he cut quite a swath among the moist coeds, but then coeds love starting rumors. In any case, there were no females attending his Forestry Engineering courses. Barney wouldn't have stood for that sort of nonsense.

We met next in 1953 on the "Operation Spruce Budworm" project, of which he had been appointed ringmaster, borrowed from the university for the anticipated few years it would take to lick this particular forest-insect problem. I was one of the few Canadian pilots on the job.

Barney arrived in a motorcade at one of the isolated gravel bush strips at the same moment that I, bored from a week of inactivity while waiting for the signal to start spraying, took off in my Stearman biplane to bash the skies with aerobatics.

"Very impressive," he said a half-hour later when I climbed from the cockpit.

"Thank you." I gave a modest smile.

"You were up there about thirty-three minutes by my watch. Any idea how much gas you burned?"

"Oh, twenty gallons maybe. Why?"

"Because, you irresponsible sonofabitch, I'm charging you for it and if I ever catch you playing that sort of game again you'll have your ass run off the project. Clear?"

In 1960 he appointed me chief pilot for the entire operation covering New Brunswick, Quebec, and Maine. Two hundred and forty aircraft based at twenty-three different airstrips. By then I had no time for games.

Although Barney has retired from active involvement in the annual forestry-spraying programs, his influence from the Canadian International Paper Company offices in the Sun Life Building is vast. The Barney Fliegers of this world never really retire: they serve as advisers, company directors, consultants or write their memoirs until dropping dead from overwork.

He walks me through the cold February air at a brisk pace to a businessman's luncheon at Madame Berger's where the only women in view wear starched aprons and accept their God-given station in life with placid equanimity made bearable by fortunes in tips. Surroundings are dark polished wood, white linen, clinking glasses, and tableware. Its patrons have homes in Westmount, N.D.G., a few live in Outremont, still fewer in Laval. René Lévesque is dementia.

"You took the train?"

Barney approves of trains. He never flies. He doesn't trust airplanes.

"I like the night train. It gives me a chance to catch up on my work without disturbing anybody."

"You're thinner."

"I'm running in front of an avalanche. Keeps me fit."

"How old are you now, Tony?"

His eyes drift for a moment; it's over a decade since he saw me last. Does he see me as his chief pilot or that jackass tumbling through the sky?

"Thirty-nine—same as Jack Benny. Funny, I used to think that was very old."

"I'm seventy," he says with wonder. "In my twenties and thirties I remember turning to the sports page first. It was the financial page during my forties and fifties. Now about all I read are the obits to see who else is gone. Hell of a way to live, waiting to die."

"Yeah, but you're looking good."

He is, too. A bit florid in the face, spiderworks of exploded capillaries purpling his cheeks and nose, but his hands and eyes are steady. Signs of a drinking man who never lost control of his habit. He reminds me of my dad. Since it's my treat he lets me order. Double scotch and sodas to clear the cobwebs.

"Cheers."

"Cheers."

An amused expression tugs his lips.

"Heard you hit the big time. Fleets of aircraft in South America, working out on the prairies, Mexico, the States. Meetings at the ministerial level. Impressive."

So he has heard already about this afternoon's meeting with the Deputy Minister of Lands and Forests. Did they phone Barney to find out if I was a crank?

"The company has grown," I agree.

"Are you making any money? If you're not, it's just so much horseshit, isn't it?"

"We're keeping our heads above water." As an afterthought I add, "I have partners."

"Working or financial?"

"Both."

"I'll give you some valuable advice. Keep your eye on the financial partners because they'll try to grab everything when the time is ripe. In the meantime, get rid of those working partners. If you don't, they'll fuck you as soon as your back is turned."

He means it. The voice of experience. But I don't try explaining the financial and corporate jigsaw of banks, private investors, personal loans, offshore bearer companies, and agreements that hold the mirage together while I race to pour concrete footings so that it will not topple.

"I need your help."

"If I can give it, it's yours. What do you want?"

"Do you know the Deputy Minister?"

"Maurice Vezina? I've spoken with him a few times. He's one of the bright ones."

"We're meeting this afternoon with his chief forester."

"So I've heard."

"When he asks for advice on the package I'm going to offer, please don't shit on me."

"I'd never do that to you, Tony. You know better than that."

"Or shit on the proposal."

"What are you offering him?"

"Four-engined passenger aircraft converted into spray planes to replace the single-engined TBMs. Instead of six hundred gallons a load at one hundred and fifty mph with a three-hundred-foot swath, these machines will carry five thousand gallons at two hundred and fifty mph with a three-thousand-foot swath at treetop level."

"Bullshit."

"Why not? The concept is sound aerodynamically and economically. Jesus, Barney, think of it! Instead of fifteen single-engine machines, five spotter planes flying on top, and a whole ground-support camp, we use one Douglas DC-seven and knock off twenty-five thousand acres an hour using fewer chemicals, getting better control, and operating with computer-precision navigation. No more errors, crashes, environmental damage, and half the price it's costing us now."

"Where are you going to get the aircraft?"

"Already got them—four old Delta Airway passenger ships sitting up in Alaska. Bought them for a song because everyone thinks they're useless. I'm moving them down to

Long Beach for conversion. The first will be licensed and flying next month. We'll do the flight testing out in the Mojave Desert at Daggett Airport. I'll be flying. First time it's ever been tried. But I want the government to turn up for the tests."

"It will never work."

"I think it will. If it doesn't, then I am full of shit but at least give me a chance to try and see what happens."

Barney sips his drink thoughtfully and looks about the room in an absent-minded fashion while he decides. One phone call when we leave Madame Berger's and Maurice Vezina's secretary will give me an apologetic smile and say that the Deputy Minister is too busy. I know how the system works.

"Tell me something. As a matter of curiosity, what are you looking for out of life?"

His conversational direction makes me blink. Is there a right or wrong answer? There can be only one reply.

"Success." Not very original, I decide.

"You mean money?"

"In part, but no—not just money. When you succeed, the money comes anyway. Like the man said: it's the scorecard to tell how well you're doing in the game."

"What then?"

He examines me in a curious way as if my answer mattered.

"Taking an idea, packaging it into a salable commodity, going out and raising money to put it together, taking it through the weeds, past the buckshot and hand grenades, making it all reality. Finally, being able to sit back and watch your creation working. Perhaps a self-satisfied smile, if no one's looking."

"That's your idea of success?"

"Sure. What else is there?"

But he won't tell his side of the story. Maybe he doesn't have one. Maybe he never found success and satisfaction, which is why he's asking me.

"What happens if you fail and everyone loses?"

"I apologize for my optimism, take an afternoon off to lick my wounds, and try something else. Not everything's a winner," I remind him unnecessarily.

"But you're satisfied this four-engined-sprayer idea will work?"

"Positive."

He spears me with his gaze, at last smiling. "Thanks for lunch."

The Deputy Minister keeps his appointment. He introduces his chief forester, Gerrard Paquet, a stocky, balding man with an intelligent face and bright, sympathetic eyes. There are others: government experts from Forestry Research, a pair of skeptical-looking Ph.D.s, and a diminutive secretary with incredible mammary development who brings everybody coffee and sticky buns.

"Bonjour, bonjour, bonjour." They have pads and pencils and have come to listen.

I'm embarrassed that we must speak in English because my French, rusty from years of disuse and impregnated with a decade of Spanish, is quite useless for a business discussion.

From my briefcase I produce charts, facts, figures, performance curves in bright, contrasting colors, trying to bowl them over with theoretical evidence of the money they will save taxpayers, the trees they will save for future generations, the environment they will save from destruction; they will become modern *coureurs de bois* and, because of their foresight and innovation, the darlings of the political arena. What I am preaching is nothing short of motherhood and my eyes glow from the sincerity of an inner flame.

There are a few questions from the pad-and-pencil crowd. Polite noncommittal smiles. They'll let me know. *"Bonjour, bonjour, bonjour."*

Supper at the Pam Pam restaurant off St. Catherine Street in downtown Montreal. Beef goulash with thick, chewy noodles and lean, crumbly beef splashed with mouth-watering gravy. Since the early 1950s I've had this love affair with the Pam Pam, driving miles out of my way when traveling to or from the East Coast, just to enjoy its specialty. I order two enormous plates of the heavily spiced goulash and later, rumbling with resonantly satisfying belches, pick my way cautiously along icy sidewalks to the hotel, where I start my evening workload.

The old Windsor Hotel retains a fragment of its former stature. Sliced, chopped in quarters, and rearranged out of consideration for real estate values, it was once the CPR bastion of Anglophone gentility and British correctness. Its rooms are vast and comfortable, the wide, carpeted hallways a wildly impractical waste of space. The atmosphere is faded Colonial elegance, a whore fighting to maintain what is left of her sagging beauty. Once, as a boy, "stopping" at the Windsor with my family during one of my father's innumerable military transfers, I remember how the morning-suited desk clerk would raise a pair of puzzled and impolite eyebrows if addressed in French. Today the reaction is the same if the staff is addressed in English.

Close to 1:00 A.M. I am sitting at the writing table in my room and hammering away on my portable typewriter, when a sudden pain knifes into my chest with an intensity and force that makes me gasp. I try belching for relief. The pain remains, sitting just under my breastbone like a great heavy stone. Indigestion? What else?

"*Avez-vous bicarbonate de soda?*" I gasp over the phone.

"*Non, m'sieu.*" The night clerk explains that the kitchen, coffee shop, and *magazin* are closed for the *nuit*. Is there something he can do to help, a bellboy to a drugstore perhaps?

"*Je suis malade.*"

"*Malade?*"

"*Oui. Malade.*"

While I'm busy trying to sort out the wording for an order of Tums or Rolaids, another, more imperious voice, comes on the phone. What is the malady from which I suffer, *s'il vous plaît?*

The French word for "heartburn" escapes me—if indeed I ever knew it. I improvise. *Brûlure* is the noun for "burn." By adding the words "sickness" and "heart," the language barrier is breached.

"*J'ai brûlure de malade coeur,*" I explain carefully.

"*Mon Dieu! Moment, m'sieu.*"

And I'm left holding an empty phone. I redial. Nothing.

Hang up and lie on the bed trying to catch my breath. It's a squeeze, this pain. Tight bands drawing tighter, tighter, tighter. I groan.

The door opens and two policemen followed by the night manager and his pimpled assistant appear at my bedside. I remain supine in my Fruit-of-the-Loom shorts, chest heaving for air. Warily the cops circle the room, peering into the drawers, the closet, at my typewriter, looking for something incriminating.

"An ambulance is on its way," the night manager says soothingly.

"It is? Why?"

Then it dawns. The silly ass has phoned the hospital. I come off the bed protesting, only to be promptly pushed horizontal by one of the alert cops.

"You don't understand. It's heartburn, not heart attack," I tell them in English.

The cop is bilingual. Everyone in Montreal is bilingual if there's an emergency.

"You 'ave de pain in de chest?"

"Yes, but it's heartburn. I need a couple of Rolaids."

"Still hurt?"

"Yes, it still hurts."

"Maybe de heart an' not de burn, eh?"

He has a point. When it comes to physical well-being, I'm as susceptible as the next man to irrational suggestion.

So maybe there is a problem with my ticker. I lie perfectly still and watch the cop frisk my pockets for ID, credit cards, money, keys. Is this legal? Is anything in Montreal? His partner opens my Samsonite, paws a few papers, and closes it. Two mustachioed and beefy ambulance men arrive wheeling a squeaking collapsible stretcher. They look like Tupamaro bandits. One sucks the trailing end of his lip hair while deciding how I'm to be transferred aboard with the minimum effort both for me and for them.

"*Bon.*" The decision is made. I'm swathed in a hotel bedsheet and wheeled away, down the lobby and through the front doors into the 30-below-zero February morning. Cold hits the sheet like a brick of ice and I begin shaking.

There's a problem with the stretcher's folding legs—left side—which refuse to fold. Much swearing *en français*. Much more shivering in English. Finally the leg collapses. I am tipped onto the pavement, then hurriedly lifted inside where both man and stretcher are strapped securely along one wall.

"Eh, Marcel. *Regardez* this one. Bad. Already his lips are *bleu*."

"*Vite, vite, vite!*"

And we're off in a cloud of powdered snow and sirens to warn the nonexistent traffic. I'm convinced now that my life can be measured in minutes. It's a race against time. The Royal Victoria Hospital sprawls near the base of Mount Royal. Faster, faster, and faster the ambulance races through vacant intersections in the glassy night, its siren whooping a portent of disaster. If there is heat in the vehicle they've hogged it all up front. I can't even move my arms. Strapped immobile like a mental incompetent. But not so immobile that I cannot shiver and breathe the freezing air or turn my head. Yet I am doomed. I feel it in my bones.

We make a screeching arrival at the hospital's emergency entrance. A half-dozen white-clads burst through the back doors and yank me out onto a gurney for a pellmell rush down a corridor, simultaneously sticking my arms with needles for blood, shaving my chest hair, tightening a pressure cuff over one bicep. At the same time there are penlight probes in each eye and stethoscope soundings by an intern who, running sideways like a crab, stumbles finally and disappears from view when he collides with the doors into cardiac emergency. I'm bordering on hysterics.

"Lie still."

I try not to blink while the ECG machine spews a ribbon of graph paper inked with wavy lines onto the floor. It is difficult not to move.

"Why are you shivering?" an angular nurse demands.

"B-b-because I'm c-c-cold."

"Nonsense! The temperature's seventy-two in here. Full climate control."

"C-c-could I have a b-b-blanket?"

"Get a blanket! He's probably in shock." The intern reappears, none the worse for his fall.

Sensible lad. Shock. Of course! Not the cold at all. I'm in shock. At once my iatrogenic symptoms take on a greater intensity until the blankets arrive. The angular nurse collects her spool of ECG paper and crosses the room to huddle with the intern and a bearded doctor with Coke-bottle lenses perched on a saber nose. Beside me, a student nurse smiles uncertainly.

"Are you in pain?"

"Do you have a Rolaid?"

In addition to my coronary problem, I'm still convinced there is the lesser pain of indigestion which, when cleared, will permit the physicians to mull over an exact diagnosis for my fluttery heart. No point in clouding the major malady with a minor ailment.

The girl fetches the conferees from across the room, relaying my request.

"What did you eat for supper?"

"Beef goulash—two plates of the stuff."

His eyes are enormous through the bottles, the pupils waver at each head movement. He orders up an antacid in a tiny paper cup which I down gratefully.

"Ahhhhhh!"

After a polite pause he asks, "Did that help?"

"Enormously."

The fires inside my chest abate. I can breathe again without pain or effort. A miracle of modern medicine.

"Hmmmm."

He stares hard at me a long time and I detect a trace of contemptuous curl to his fur-shadowed lips.

"Your ECG is normal."

"Really? Well, that is good to hear." And I sit up, prepared to discuss the diagnosis further.

"What do you do for a living?"

"My job? I'm in business—airplanes, money, that sort of thing. My heart is all right then? I mean, you're absolutely certain I didn't have a heart attack? There must be something else you should check."

"You fly airplanes?"

"Yes, I do. Seems to me I read about a blood test for enzymes."

"Which company do you fly for?"

"My own company."

I don't want to rise from the gurney wrapped in a sheet, forced to make my own way back to the hotel in a taxi at this hour if there's any possibility of hanging around until after breakfast.

"Big airplanes or small?" The doctor's a frustrated pilot.

"Four engines."

"I've always wanted to fly. They wouldn't take me in the air force because of my eyes, you know. Need twenty/twenty in both eyes."

"Ah well, doctor, you didn't miss much."

"You were in the air force?" He makes it sound as if I'd escorted the Magi.

"Back in the Fifties. I was very young." I tell him apologetically. "My heart, doctor, it was indigestion, wasn't it?"

"Maybe."

He decides to keep me under observation a few days as a precaution.

"How few? I mean, there are appointments I have to keep. Meetings to attend."

"Two or three days—say three."

They give me a private room on the cardiac floor with telephone, television, and telephoto winter view of the white and black, ice and glass city.

There's a timeless quality to Montreal. The warmhearted old dowager of the mountain is destined to live forever, a polyglot of children at her skirts: French, Greek, Hebrew, English, German, Italian, Portuguese. She has many faces, is many things, and French is only a part. It is the country's only true melting pot, and no matter how hard developers try to emulate the stark sterility and trick rectangular realism of Toronto and Calgary or Edmonton, this old dowager will remain the queen of graceful cities.

I sleep fitfully until the day lifts bright and clear from a brittle rosy dawn. After breakfast and a change of linen—"But, nurse, I've only been in bed two and a half hours"—I call home and tell Helen not to worry because it's just indigestion.

"Then why are they keeping you in hospital?"

Good question. An hour could be spent exploring the possibilities but there isn't time. I've an appointment with Curtis Fincham of Canadair Limited at 10:00 A.M. to discuss a five-year spraying program in Tunisia. All the figures are in my briefcase. Somehow I have to get the hotel to send it over to the hospital with my clothes or I'm lost. No phone numbers, no charts, no records. Business emasculation.

Peter Cheeseman, one of my partners, is in Kenai, Alaska, with a crew readying the DC-7s for ferry to Long Beach, California. Eric Schwendau, another partner, is down in Managua overseeing our Central American operations and trying to keep Dino from soaring off into the abyss and plunging the company into financial disaster. Marcos Vilela, our Brazilian partner, is howling again for more aircraft and money to keep the tiny operation at São Joaquim do Barra afloat. There is another investors' meeting in Toronto tonight, a payroll to meet, three bank managers needing their tummies rubbed, and I'm due in Los Angeles the day after tomorrow. I'm Mr. Fixit.... I did not make a conscious effort to acquire business responsibilities. They evolved through circumstances.

After returning to Canada in 1965 I gave up flying because of severe chemical poisoning. The chemical endrin—now almost universally banned—was used to control tobacco hornworm in southwestern Ontario. A chlorinated hydrocarbon of the DDT family, although many times more lethal, the product attacks the cortex of the central nervous system in animals, insects, and humans. An ounce of pure endrin ingested through skin, mouth, or lungs will produce convulsions and death within an hour for the average-sized human, a half-day for cattle and horses. On insects, the stuff is practically instantaneous.

Mixed at a pint per gallon of water, the resulting mix is sprayed on tobacco crops at a half-gallon an acre. But someone forgot to add the water to my mixing tank and I flew out with a tank full of pure endrin. The last time this was tried as an experiment for ultra-low volume spraying, the pilot died.

Chemical poisoning is insidious in its invasion of the body. First, there's a light euphoria and loss of motor function affecting the fine-tuning mechanisms of sight, balance, and muscular coordination. Next comes dizziness, nausea, soaring heart rate, vomiting, convulsions, and death.

Recognizing the symptoms, I found a vacant hay field close to a farmhouse and landed promptly. The bottom of the aircraft was awash with endrin. A seal on the shut-off valve had ruptured, spraying the cockpit with a fine mist of lethal poison. Because of my face-mask respirator I hadn't smelled the gut-wrenching odor. Body absorption had taken place through my clothing.

I staggered drunkenly to the farmhouse where the owner graciously drove me into the nearest hospital at Tillsonburg in his pickup. Upon arrival at emergency I was told ungraciously to take a seat and wait.

Unless I was prepared to die awaiting my turn, something dramatic had to be done. I reached across the reception counter and tore away the duty nurse's shirt front and bra.

"Pick up a pencil and start writing. I have only minutes before going into convulsions and then it will be too late. Phone Poison Control Centre in Toronto and ask for Dr. Mastramateo. Tell him you have a spray pilot with dermal endrin poisoning."

To her everlasting credit, she managed to get it all down along with the phone number while standing bare-breasted in that crowded reception room and in consequence saved my life.

The next thing I remember is swimming into a dizzy consciousness miles away in London, Ontario, at another Victoria Hospital to which I'd been ambulanced.

Recovery took ages. For a while I lost both the power of coherent speech and the ability to stand upright unassisted. Plagued by nauseous vertigo and blinding headaches, I toyed with suicide, laying elaborate plans in order to make look like an accident so that Helen could collect on the double-indemnity clause of my insurance. Yet when the time arrived for putting my plot into action, I realized suddenly that these plans had been the first rational thoughts of which I'd been capable in weeks, and decided accordingly that recovery was just around the corner. And so it was, but oh God, it took a long, long time.

Summer changed to fall, fall into winter, and it was not until the following spring that I dared to venture solo from the house or to drive a car. My flying days were over. Any thought of climbing into an aircraft cockpit made me break out in a cold sweat and relive the symptoms of my Waterloo. Like an AA member, odors of cleaning fluid, exhaust fumes, paints, and insecticides brought about a violent reaction for months afterward.

What an amazing creation is the human mind—able to call up from memory and duplicate the sorrows, horrors, and physical impairments long cured and assumed forgotten. To this day the smell of some insecticides and cleaning compounds makes me ill.

Five years passed. I acquired a handsome son, two beautiful daughters, a big new house with heated pool and miniscule mortgage, plus a quarter-acre of lawn to mow. It came through hard work, good credit, and long hours spent developing an industrial idea for curing tobacco using a pressure heat principle and new kiln design. With 150,000 acres of the weed in southwestern Ontario, Quebec, and the Maritimes, there was no shortage of sales. Even giant Imperial Tobacco bought twelve units for their new experimental farm in Prince Edward Island. Money rolled in.

I never looked at an airplane nor felt any inclination to climb into a cockpit. It had become a pleasurable memory from youth and I considered myself lucky to have survived. Besides, the foreign scene had changed. No longer did Latin American countries welcome itinerant pilots, preferring to use their own who, after many tragic accidents and wrecked aircraft, had begun to learn the art of keeping their machines intact and themselves alive.

One hot summer day in 1970 Peter Cheeseman came to visit me. A stocky Yorkshireman with dark, straight hair, square chin, and startlingly bright blue eyes, he operated a small repair and overhaul depot near the village of Norwich. Years before, I'd used his single grass strip as the main maintenance base for my local operations. Besides being a damn good mechanic prepared to work any hour of the day or night in an emergency, Cheeseman never gouged his customers. He had six kids, a happy wife, an even disposition, and dreams of glory.

"I need help," he began, chewing a dead cigar.

On hot summer afternoons I paddled around my pool on a chair-raft with a cold drink on one armrest and a telephone trailing thirty feet of cord on the other. My manufacturing interests had been sold and I'd been dabbling in real estate speculation and the mortgage market. There's a certain delight in sitting back and watching your money multiply virtually unaided. At least until boredom sets in and one is ripe for change. I was ripe.

"You need money?"

"I always need money. But no, that's not why I came. I need answers and you're the only one I know smart enough to have them."

Score one for Cheeseman. The first rule of salesmanship is never to approach the sucker head on for his money. Use the oblique approach. Soften him up. Ask his advice. Everybody feels flattered being asked to advise. Pump his ego up to 100 psi. When he's been flattered, patted, and had his ears scratched, chances are you won't have to ask for a thing because he'll offer whatever you want.

Curiosity aroused, I paddled over to hear more. "Have a drink?"

He's a scotch-and-water man. No ice. His problem was the amalgamation of two bankrupt aviation companies with his marginally profitable maintenance operation: two losers dragging down a winner. The price of unprofitable expansion based on unwarranted optimism.

"But I have a way out. A Montreal company has an inside track on a multimillion-dollar spraying contract in Tunisia. They've asked me to help price it."

"Why you?"

Peter Cheeseman isn't exactly a household name in the aviation industry as a mechanic or consultant.

"Because I registered our company name with CIDA. It came as a referral."

Smart move. The Canadian International Development Agency gives away close to a billion a year in foreign aid, some of the money to countries that actually need it for projects that actually work. But for the most part, businessmen regard CIDA as a political scandal and national disgrace. A milch cow to be teated during periods of economic recession and to provide cushy sinecures for Liberal party faithful.

"What type of aircraft?"

"I don't know. You can decide that after reading the specs."

"How sure is this contract?"

"One hundred percent."

If he believed that, he'd believe anything. From a tatty plastic zipper case he produced an assortment of maps, aerial photographs, and impressive computer printouts, the latter courtesy of Canadair Limited of Montreal who were interested in selling their behemoth water bombers as agricultural sprayers. The computer assessment proved that their CL-215 would be the ideal machine for Tunisia. Naturally.

The middleman company in this venture was operated by Curtis Fincham, a former air force colonel and sales vice-president for Canadair. It bore the exotic name of NAREMCO, standing for Natural Resources Energy Management Company. High-voltage stuff.

I pawed through the information, intrigued by its scope and bottom-line numbers. If such an operation could be organized, financed, equipped, and transported successfully to Tunisia, the participants could retire comfortably on the tax-free returns. The CIDA guidelines, written by somebody with only the vaguest idea of what might be required, were outlined in very general abstract terms.

A monarch butterfly flitted above the emerald water, dodging tiny predators or darting after insects. Which? The air was humid and hazy, redolent with perfume from my rose garden. Children screeched happily nearby.

In retrospect, and with the clarity of hindsight, what I should have done was fold everything away into the tatty case, express polite interest in his efforts, and offer a loan for a piece of the action. Being a stubborn Yorkshireman, he'd have refused, finished his drink, and departed—and I wouldn't have wound up with a decade of problems and a heart attack. But hindsight is always twenty/twenty. Instead of using my head, I followed my heart and dove back into the aviation business with a vengeance.

First step on the road back came with reinstating my pilot's license. The bureaucracy responsible for aviation matters believe that pilots forget everything in five years, so all medicals, written exams, and flight tests have to be redone. Fortunately it's like riding a bicycle, or sex: once learned to proficiency never forgotten. By first snow I had an airline transport rating in a snappy new leather folder and was trying to sort out the corporate mess that was Midair Aviation Limited of Norwich, Ontario.

The company had four single-engine crop-spraying aircraft, a modest overhaul shop, an asthmatic pickup truck, and $150,000 of debt. In 1970 that was a lot of bread. Receivables were a few overdue accounts from disgruntled tobacco farmers, and whatever business could be promoted for the shop. By Christmas I had sunk too much time and money into the disaster to walk away. Since CIDA would take months to make a decision on the Tunisian spraying proposal there was ample time to expand the company's horizons.

A fast four-seat aircraft was borrowed and we flew to Las

Vegas for the annual international agricultural aviation convention. Cheeseman was entranced. There were delegates from around the world. For the first time he saw work potential beyond the three-month Canadian season. A Brazilian delegation attended, headed by Dr. Marcos Vilela, a young quadrilingual spray pilot with a Ph.D. from the University of São Paulo. He worked with the Coffee Institute and claimed that hundreds of aircraft were needed to combat the spread of coffee leaf rust, a fungus infection threatening to ruin Brazil's coffee-export future. Would we be interested in visiting the country for a first-hand inspection of the problem with the objective of opening a South American operation? We certainly would.

A month later we leased an eight-place executive twin, which I flew to Brazil and the summer of the south: Belém on the Amazon, Recife, Rio de Janeiro, and São Paulo, inland to the Mato Grosso, where a few ranches are larger than some European nations.

There were five of us on board the aircraft and, after two months' examination, the opinion was unanimous. Brazil needed a thousand aircraft, a thousand trained pilots, a thousand problems solved. But it was a military dictatorship where despite crowings of equality and common sense, a brutal bureaucracy bumbled for months over the simplest decisions.

Vilela, our new partner and chief executive officer of the newly formed Midair do Brazil, promised to smooth the way for importation permissions on the aircraft we would send. Cheeseman wanted twenty. Vilela insisted on thirty. I figured if we could dig up financing for five we would be working miracles. We flew home to Canada in time to meet the spring.

A race for money began. Neither governments nor conventional lending institutions were interested in bankrupt aviation companies, regardless of their exotica, so I turned to private investors and a professional financial analyst to make it hang together. A half-million dollars was needed for starters.

Eric Schwendau was my age and a self-made millionaire who operated a financial consultant service in London. He heard my story and began to vibrate at the long-term prospects.

By July, Midair was solvent with over a quarter-million new capital from private lenders, including personal resources, family friends, and relations. Anyone who ropes his relations into a business deal has got to be an evangelist.

From across the country spray aircraft were leased and operated under the Midair logo: prairie wheat, Quebec forests, East Coast potatoes, Ontario farmlands and orchards. By season's peak, twenty-eight machines were working.

Additionally, 90 percent financing on eight new aircraft for Brazil was promised through the U.S. Export Bank, all of it arranged by Eric and North American Rockwell, the aircraft manufacturer. I returned to Brazil, this time on the airlines, to set up the Rio office, visit the customers in the interior, and stopped off at Managua on my way home to see Dino Zaglaviras. Lease arrangements were made for all his aircraft to join us in Brazil after the spray season in Nicaragua.

Back in Canada, the money continued to roll in. A few disgruntled investors from the original Midair mess tried a company take-over, but it was quickly quashed and Eric was elected president unanimously.

In the flush of October's anticipation for success, it seemed incredible that by the New Year everything had ground to a halt. What appeared so easy, suddenly became impossible.

In a fit of pique against anything Canadian, U.S. Secretary of the Treasury John Connolly refused to allow Export Bank financing. Zaglaviras lost half his aircraft fleet through foolish accidents. Vilela lost one of his two for the same reason and, although buried under three million dollars' worth of contract work, had been unable to obtain from his government permission to bring in more than one foreign-owned aircraft and pilot. The idiocy of nationalism. Our world had crumbled about our heads.

A few days after the New Year I held a wake at the company office in Norwich to formulate an approach to use with our shareholders in explaining what had happened and whether salvage from bankruptcy was possible. Something was needed to spark investor confidence. Something tangible.

Cheeseman produced a current edition of Trade-a-plane, an aviation sales magazine. In it four Douglas DC-7 aircraft were advertised for sale in Kenai, Alaska. Originally owned by Delta Airlines, they had been equipped with 5,000-gallon tankage and used for hauling fuel oil to Alaska's north slope while Atlantic Richfield put together their cracking plant at Prudhoe Bay.

"Wouldn't they make one hell of a sprayer?" he mused.

"They certainly will," I said. "What's the owner's phone number?"

And we were off and running again. . . .

On the third morning of my stay at the Royal Victoria Hospital, Barney Flieger phones to express sympathy and inquire on progress.

"A false alarm," I tell him. "They're booting me out today."

"Good. You're too young for a coronary. Supposed to be for old bastards like me."

"Amen."

"By the way, I spoke to Maurice Vezina. The government have decided to give your four-engined idea a try. Prove that it works and they'll have a million-dollar contract for you this summer."

I am stunned. Reprieve! Phoenix rising from the ashes.

"Did you hear what I said?"

"Yes. Thanks, Barney."

"For what? It was their decision. I told them you were full of shit."

How swiftly a decade passes in the pursuit of success.

Kingston, Canada

20 January 1980

My first walk outside the room is along the hospital's busy corridors. Coronary rehabilitation. Slow, slippered steps to the double fire doors, a judicious pause for breath while leaning against the wall, then a cautious return to the room for recovery from this gigantic effort.

At any moment I expect the nurses to charge out from their secret places with a wheelchair because I've overtaxed myself and the red light above their monitor is flashing preparatory to my demise. But no, I make it back without incident and Mr. Sung beams his approval.

"You better."

"I'm tired."

A week has passed. My survival odds now are overwhelming, equal to recovery from a bad bout of flu. I sit in our visitor's chair waiting for the damaged muscle to stop racing.

Incredible how we gallop through life ignoring our heart, taking its functioning for granted, never a thought to what is happening to it. Those chest-heaving exertions at labor, the steady thrumming when headaches press the brain, that drumbeat in our ears when slipping into the catacombs of sleep, and the palpitations of love—or lust—each a message from our heart: "Hey, man! I'm in here and I'm working."

Only when it pains or fails us do we notice this muscular miracle within our breasts.

Consider the marvel of performance: every hour pumping enough blood to fill a pair of forty-five-gallon barrels, over two thousand gallons each day. And, if we are lucky enough to attain our biblical allotment of threescore and ten, by life's end this fist-sized muscle will have pumped an incredible fifty-two million gallons. Thirteen hundred railway tank cars stretching to the horizons. Such analogies are mind-boggling.

An oversolicitous matron with violet hair rinse and ample thighs wheels a trolley load of books into the room and berths alongside my chair.

"And how long have we been here?" she gushes.

"A week," I mumble.

"Are we feeling better?"

"We are."

"And I imagine we'll be going home soon, won't we?"

Anything is possible. Hospitals attract do-gooders. KC Women's Auxiliary, Salvation Army, Junior Baptist Helpers, Christian Temperance Union, Junior League, everyone with a mission to succor his fellow men and women sooner or later appears at the door. For some they are no doubt a Godsend, but to me they are a pain in the neck and I wish they'd stay home or at church or wherever they come from. I want to enjoy my illness without interruption.

When I was younger and healthier, when death and illness were merely words, I used to think how pleasurable it would be to depart this life to the strains of music. Dvořák's New World Symphony, perhaps, or the temple duet from "The Pearl Fishers." Even the romanticism of Tchaikovsky's Overture to "Romeo and Juliet" would be acceptable. Surrounded by friends, loved ones, and the soaring chords of musical genius, I would expire with a smile in the best Hollywood tradition.

But reality turns out to be quite different. Nothing is more annoying during illness than to be pestered continually by well-wishers, do-gooders, faith healers, and soprano-voiced children. Music likewise becomes an annoyance. Tunes are noise; melodic chords nothing more than a cacophony of grating, mismatched notes.

The flabby matron with the violet rinse has a whisky rasp to her voice. Pebbles on gravel. Mr. Sung is ignored as though he didn't exist. I want to trade places with him so that I can watch the intrusion instead of participating.

"I recommend these to all my heart patients. Good solid stuff. Thought-provoking. Exceptional."

Her supply of adjectives exhausted for the moment, she

plucks two volumes from the top shelf of her literary wagon to thrust into my lap. Are there books for the burn victims farther along the hall? Encouraging volumes for cancer patients on the next floor? What does she advocate for the neurological crowd?

A file card is produced for me to sign with her ballpoint.

"Now then, if we leave hospital before I return we will be sure to remember to leave our books at the nurses' desk, won't we?"

I assure her that we will and am awarded the "I knew I could trust you" eye-lock before she wheels away.

The books have been written by M.D.s. Fatuous commentaries packed with bromides designed to alleviate fears of future sex life, family problems, social adjustment, reinstatement of employment: "What the boss will think when you return to the office," plus all sorts of good, sensible, straight-from-the-shoulder advice. Don't smoke, stay slim, exercise daily, avoid stress, and above all keep happy and think positive. Wahoo!

The pages are well thumbed, corners bent, whole paragraphs of silly prose underlined in frantic red ballpoint. Since neither author experienced a coronary, I find their advice both obvious and suspect. There is an oblique reference to the patient's next heart attack. Oh yeah?

Common sense tells me that there has got to be another next week, next month, next year—sometime. It's like the inevitability of nuclear war. Not the same heart attack of course. That portion of the organ affected by this attack has died already and healing over with scar tissue. Next time a different part will die. Maybe all of it. Exercise daily, they state. I get to my feet and shuffle off.

In the room next door is a charming man in his seventies. Mr. Leader is tall and stooped, a stonemason with hard, solid hands and a gentle disposition. He operates a rock quarry, making gravestones—heavy heartbreaking work. He's back in hospital with his third attack.

When I introduce myself he gets up from his chair to

shake hands and inquire politely after my health. Three heart attacks. How much stress is there in making monuments? Surely time limits cannot apply. How could there be deadlines to meet? He doesn't smoke, drink, or eat anything to make a dietitian frown, and works like a Clydesdale. Three heart attacks?

"First one come eleven years back," he explains in a soft, apologetic tone, surprised at my interest because cardiac patients tend to be self-centered. "Then a second come along two years back. Couldn't lift much after that. Had to hire a young feller because my nephew don't like the business. Hard to find young people willing to work nowadays. Guess I should have retired when I was ahead, eh?"

Monuments have been his life—stone angels, gothic script, miniature obelisks. He's never had a wife or family, never known close "touch and feel" affection, only an adventurous nephew who "run off to join the Marines, for gosh sakes. Can you imagine that? A foreign army!" he exclaims sadly as if a world of madness had swept away all common sense while he'd been chipping stone.

His last attack came a few days after mine. A mild coronary, so they told him. So insignificant that it wasn't necessary to put him into the fishbowl of intensive care.

"But they don't know. Not really. Doctors never tell a feller anything. I got a feeling this time things is just about over for me. Ever had that feeling?"

"Every morning for the past week."

He rewards me with a chuckle. "But you're young. You'll get over it."

I'm young? The wrong end of my forties and oblivion a decade or two away and this charmer thinks I'm young. Everything is relative. My children think I'm an antique. Antediluvian in attitude and musical appreciation. Charles De Gaulle once said that old age was a shipwreck. I feel as if I'm rushing onto a lee shore.

"You'll get over it, too," I promise professionally.

"Don't think so. Not this time."

And I slipper out, leaving him staring wistfully at the winter rooftops. Is there a prescience of doom granted each of us as the fateful day approaches?

Another rest. Gradually my heart slows its thumpings. Two student nurses turn up to change the bedclothes. Bright cherub-cheeked girls in their late teens for whom mortality is still a textbook word and nursing a purity of selfless purpose. At what age do we grow wise like Mr. Sung?

"You try again?" he inquires.

He isn't allowed out of bed and, although he hasn't had a heart attack, suffers continually from angina. His doctor is playing musical pills, endeavoring to find a tablet combination to ease his problem. There is, of course, no ultimate cure but death. Two nights ago an angina crept into our room and under his sheets to seize him while he slept. A cowardly attack. I rang for the duty nurse because he had become too paralyzed with pain to find the button.

"Once more to the end of the hall," I announce and shuffle off.

"Good to keep the heart working. Sure."

I don't know how good it is but it's certainly exhausting. Lordy, I feel like one of those poor doddering antiques that one sees creeping vacantly about on lush green lawns at an old folks' home. Just now I am frightfully conscious of age, seeing my hourglass with less than a third of its sand remaining and still running through the narrow opening, still piling success and failure in a tiny pyramid of gritty memories.

Quite by accident I learn that Mr. Sung is eighty-four. Incredible. He doesn't look a day over fifty-five. We were talking of the early years before the war. In my memory's mists THE WAR was World War II, but Mr. Sung had been speaking of World War I. The Great War.

He'd arrived steerage from mainland China in the summer of 1913 and found a job washing dishes in a Chinese restaurant for twenty-five cents a day and a pallet in the attic. A fortune.

In those days not so very long ago, Orientals were forbidden citizenship or permission to bring their families to

Canada's deserted shores. A matter of racial purity designed to keep the True North Strong and Free—and White.

"So what's wrong with that? Ever look at Australia's laws? I mean they just don't let in Chinks and darkies. Once these birds get a foot in the door, next thing you know all their aunts, uncles, brothers, sisters, and in-laws turn up on welfare and it's standing room only. And they breed like rabbits, y'know."

Unofficial word from an immigration officer whose father, a tailor from Sardinia, saved half a lifetime to get to America so that his son could be born in a land of opportunity.

"I mean look at Genghis Khan and guys like that. If they get a chance they'll take over the whole fucking world."

Yeah.

His aunts, uncles, and grandparents still remember their island, but told me they would never go back. Not even for a visit.

When Mr. Sung arrived, he knew he *had* to go back. Chinese were second-class visitors, regarded by government and citizenry as slave labor to be used and discarded. Sad. Even sadder the treadmill on which they found themselves after a few years of hard work in the restaurant or laundry business.

"So what happened to all the Chinese laundries?"

Mr. Sung smiles. "Old people work laundry. Grow old and die. Children go to university. Learn business, medicine, law. Buy automatic washers and dryers. No more Chinese laundries. Starch companies go broke. Very unhappy time."

There is humor behind his twinkling eyes. The restaurant business is different, every Chinaman his own maitre d'. Start with nothing. Work sixteen hours a day for ten years and you have your own place complete with paper lanterns plus enough money for passage back to China to find a wife. From then on it's a visit every five years to see how much your kids have grown, how much your wife has aged, and if you can make her pregnant again before the *Empress* sails from Shanghai.

Sometimes when he arrived back to his business he'd find that the man left in charge had robbed him blind or simply closed the doors and run off to open his own establishment in the next town. He would have to start all over with new dishes, new pots, new paper lanterns. In 1947 the government changed the rules, decreeing that Chinese men with Chinese wives could live together as God intended. The Age of Enlightenment.

His wife is eighty-two. She comes every day before noon and again soon after supper. A spry, elfin woman with smooth features and neatly tied gray hair, she arrives carrying a shopping bag filled with knitting, clean pajamas, slippers, and Chinese newspapers. She never learned English. "Hello, good-by, thank you," but that's all.

I give up my chair—her chair really—and go sit on the bed.

"Oh, thank you." She smiles.

There's great comfort sharing accommodation in hospital, particularly when you know that the chap in the next bed is worse off than you. His experiences and misery provide a yardstick for your own progress. Or is it now a meterstick by government legislation?

Truly, misery loves company. Not to share but rather to compare. For one it becomes the measurement of progress, for the other the distance yet to be traveled. For the seriously ill, accommodation in a crowded ward must be nirvana.

I know that Mr. Sung is much sicker than I. At eighty-four how many grains are left in the top half of his hourglass. Whichever of my arteries narrowed and plugged, the damage is done. Irreparably. But the angina is gone. In retrospect, I prefer a minor heart attack to constant angina. A fair exchange. A dicky heart can be babied in comfort with a clear mind while the rest of the body still has an ability to enjoy the sensual pleasures of food, sound, sight, smell, walking, sex.

But for someone bullied by angina, every move must be planned in advance. Not to eliminate the pain because that never happens, but to adjust the mind to the anticipated level of pain coincident with a specific action. Walks must be slow and short, stairs taken one at a time with long pauses for rest; meals must be light and sparse, every action slow and methodical. Sex is quite impossible.

Mr. Sung's angina comes with no movement at all. A fast-paced dream and he'll awake gasping the way I did a few weeks ago. The question is, how many of his arteries are narrowing? Many or one? If only one, is it a critical one? Solution comes with guesswork and a game of pills.

"Not true." Dr. Rice informs me. He's Koval's stand-in when the great man is not in residence. A handsome young lad with wavy brown hair and semiserious blue eyes, he makes me feel old. His visits are unaccompanied, which, in the pecking order, means he's a junior.

"We can do angiography. Photography inside the heart and all its connecting arteries. Actually pinpoint where the problem lies."

He says it proudly, as though he had a finger in the discovery.

"Then, if it's warranted, we can go in and perform a by-pass to get the blood flowing around the problem area."

By-pass. I'd heard the expression before. Open-heart surgery. It has taken medicine five thousand years to advance that half-inch behind the breastbone and be able to fix heart valves, leaky arteries, blockages, to install pacemakers or even a new heart.

"Then why not take a peek inside poor old Mr. Sung?"

"He's an old man," Rice says, not unkindly. "Even with an angiogram there are risks. He could have an infarct during the examination."

"Thereby spoiling somebody's record? Did you ever consider maybe he'd prefer that to the pain? Has anyone asked what he thinks?"

"It's not that simple. Even if we find his trouble and could correct it surgically, we can't operate. The age limit is seventy. It used to be sixty."

Catch 22. When patients are too old to be saved.

"But look at the man. He looks sixty. And who the hell decided arbitrarily that seventy would be the cut-off point?"

"Surgeons make their own policies. Besides, he wouldn't survive major surgery, believe me. It's the last attempt to cure any problem. Until then we try everything else."

"But if everything else doesn't work and it's too late for surgery because you frittered away your time experimenting, what then?"

"The patient dies."

"How does it feel playing God?"

"I know it sounds unfair, but it isn't if you stop and think about it. Wouldn't you agree that it's better to operate on someone whose survival odds are greater than an eighty-four-year-old man's?"

"You mean like me?"

"Like you."

"I don't know, doctor. I've never played God."

We speak softly, keeping our voices below the level of musical Chinese conversation from the next bed. Rice looks at Mr. Sung with compassion. He means it when he says: "The best we can do for him now is make him comfortable and hope to hell one of the dosages will relieve his problem. Yet, speaking practically, how much more life can an eighty-four-old man expect?"

I don't know the answer but it is certainly food for thought. Are there radical differences between the quality of medicine in socialized-health-care countries and nations like the United States, where virtually everything is cash on the barrelhead unless you're part of an insurance program or charity case stuffed into an overcrowded county hospital?

Putting aside the few doctors who are in it strictly for the money, and patients who are in hospitals strictly for imaginary ailments, how much difference is there in the quality of care between hospitals, between doctors, between nations? Does the Hippocratic Oath alter between national boundaries and hospital boards? Is there unspoken agreement between physicians to set healing priorities according to age, illness, or financial consideration, and pull the plug when pain and suffering reach a point beyond what the Creator intended? I hope so. But I don't envy those that must make the decision.

"Most heart troubles stem from the coronary arteries," Dr. Rice explains, sketching me a beautiful diagram. He should have been a draftsman. "As they thicken and narrow with age, blood supply to the heart is reduced, and the heart muscle becomes weaker from the lack of blood. A thrombosis, or clot, in one of these arteries can be mildly uncomfortable or killing, depending upon where it happens, which artery or subartery is affected.

"According to your electrocardiogram the damage is in the upper left side, at the back of your heart muscle. You're a lucky man. Your blockage took place in a secondary coronary artery, not a primary. Your angina came as the blood flow was squeezed from providing nourishment to that part of the heart. But before the blockage became total, hundreds of small capillaries started taking over the load, in a sense turning themselves into new veins and arteries to feed your heart."

"But not enough to prevent an attack."

"True, but enough extra help so that only moderate damage was done. Without that backup you might not be with us. It happens."

He tells of two cases that never reached hospital, men younger than I. The first was hanging drapery track for his wife when he fell over dead. The second was a health nut and avid jogger who died in his shorts and Nikes during the first mile of his regular evening run. Jogging, for Christ sake.

But these are unusual. Normally there are warnings: shortness of breath, general tiredness—and angina. Yet everybody loves to shudder when he hears of the airline captain who climbed off his 747 and into his Olds and dropped dead in the parking lot. True. Or the insurance examination by two eminent physicians, both of whom pronounced the applicant sound as The Rock, only to have him die in the elevator on his way out of the building. True.

"But those are the exception, not the rule. In your case the rule applied. Angina, coronary, recovery. Your scar tissue is healing, but ten percent of your heart is gone forever, so the remaining part must take up the load."

"Until another artery plugs. How much do I lose then? Another ten percent, or can you guarantee no more than twenty-five percent? I mean, if one has plugged up, there must be others waiting in line saying 'Me too!' I feel like a time bomb."

He likes my sense of humor, but I wasn't trying to be funny. Can't he understand how it feels? Did I at his age? Of course not. Doctor or not, he dwells in the invincible twenties, where everyone lives forever and all the dead become cadavers, medical curiosities to be dissected and probed, and where all the sick of the world are patients to be treated according to current medical philosophy. I can't blame him. His hiatus of immortality will pass.

"Why can't we do one of those angio things and find out if anything else is close to shut-off?"

"Angiogram. We can, but not immediately after an attack. Give it a few months until your heart settles down and you've recovered your strength. There are risks in an angiogram, too, you know," he reminds me again.

"Doctor, there are risks in using a bedpan, but it does wonders for your peace of mind."

He leaves laughing. I feel depressed. It's foolish, I know, when there's so much for which to be thankful. Everyone needs a stay in hospital to appreciate the gift of life. All society's horrors are on parade.

The survivor of that seven-second highway holocaust in living color on the evening news, translated into months of skin grafts, plastic surgery, enduring indescribable pain and suffering. His eyes regard me through hollow cores of anguish when I drop by the Burn Room.

Without skin, at least on the upper torso, arms, and part of his face, the poor man lies naked, floating on a bed of tiny glass beads supported by air. The intricate webbing of surface muscles and denuded flesh appear pinkish-blue and very dry, like venison. Damp medicinal cloths cloak the destruction. Moisture is the key to his survival. Over the months ahead, pieces of skin from his back and legs will be transferred to rebuild the skinless portions of his body. He needs skin to breathe.

I try a few words of comfort. He looks at me uncomprehendingly. Then his nurse appears and shoos me out the door. In the hall she explains that the man is an Italian immigrant, a cement worker. Less than two years in the country, he was on his honeymoon in a new car with an illegal driver's license because he couldn't pass the test. His wife didn't make it.

The twenty-five-year three-pack-a-day man squeaks by, pushing his oxygen bottle. A wheezing cadaver with one lung removed, the other crippled by emphysema, he is destined to end his days tethered to a plastic tube. He stops to talk and I learn that despite the gray wispy hair and sunken cheeks he's ten years younger than I.

"Have you quit?" he gasps.

"Quit what?"

"Smoking."

"Yes. I've been clean for a week," I tell him righteously.

"Miss it?"

"No. In fact until you brought the subject up, I hadn't even thought about it."

"Jesus, I miss it! Tried a couple of drags last week and nearly choked to death. God, it felt good. Know what I mean?"

Not really. Maybe he has a death wish. Welcome to Marlboro Country. I feel better already. A lightness in my step.

My son Peter visits me each weekday after school. He is thirteen and in grade seven. He comes alone, preferring to leave the evenings for his sisters and mother when he says the room gets too crowded and there are never enough chairs. Actually, I think he enjoys secretly this opportunity of doing something completely on his own instead of going home where he is condemned to the company of women.

He is at that awkward age, still too young to discuss things with his mother in adult terms and too old now to play with his sisters. He needs his father and I'm afraid I haven't been around much these past years to give him what he needed most of all: my time.

No one asked him to come and I'm certain there are more

pressing matters than walking three miles each way in bitter cold to see me. I feel guilt like a character from an Ibsen play, filled with emotional layers of contradictions. The novelty of visiting me I was sure would wear off. But it didn't, and now I look forward to his visits, even saving sandwiches and crackers from the huge meal trays I order each noon so that I'll have something to hand him when he arrives. His appetite is ravenous. A joy to watch.

He appears shortly after four, rosy-cheeked and still a little breathless from his walk. I envy his health, his young heartbeat quickening to the tempo of life. With my features and his mother's placid temperament, his is proof of the dichotomy of genes within a family. We play cards, sometimes chess or backgammon, and talk. For me the games are unimportant because it is his conversation upon which I thrive.

Quite suddenly I have discovered how important the children have become to me. A passport to immortality, as I have been for my father and his father before him. When all's said and done, my children will be the only tangible evidence I shall leave behind to prove that I walked this earth, loved, and was loved.

In the early years, when we participate in the miracle of birth and hold their tiny bodies tremblingly in our gigantic hands and gaze in fascination at the screaming or sleeping products we helped to create, it is difficult to regard them as human. They are products of our motherhood or manhood, brought about through the natural order of things—objects to love, care for, clean, and feed. Certainly not human—at least not then.

For fathers, children are playthings provided to ease the cares of daily work and frustrations encountered in the world of wages, salaries, and commissions. Ten, perhaps fifteen, inspirational minutes are devoted to offspring, after which the evening paper, supper, or television takes precedence. Or, in my case, disappearing into my study behind closed doors to spend the rest of the evening formulating business developments, pretending all the time that I am doing it for my family.

Bullshit.

I do it for myself, completely selfish motivation driving me to achieve more, acquire more, know more, succeed more, and so enjoy the accolades of well-deserved recognition from my peers. Such vanity. Such stupidity. Such a misplaced sense of values.

In a thunderbolt of comprehension it had come to me that nothing is more important than helping fulfill my children's expectations, while at the same time trying to guide their inquiring minds along the paths of knowledge, teaching them to question everything, accept nothing as fact until they have satisfied themselves to what is truth. Then be prepared to stand firm with that belief. A tall order.

Peter lost a year of schooling when we lived in California. Athletics was the only mandatory subject at Costa Mesa's Tewinkle Junior High School. As an *out-of-stater* with a funny accent and gray socks, he was branded immediately as a fag, was regularly beaten up, and had his bicycle stolen all within the first few weeks. Finally, after several long, and apparently persuasive, talks with his mother, he decided to fight back, picked the biggest of his tormenters, and knocked him on his ass. After that he joined the swimming team and began winning ribbons. No one bothered him again. But he learned little or nothing at the school except how to duck a right cross, hold his temper in check when confronted with stupidity, and keep his mouth shut. All useful knowledge on the road of life but of little academic value. What little he did manage to learn that year his mother taught him.

Where was I? Off chasing rainbows, flying home for recuperative weekends, maintaining the nodding acquaintance with my family developed so masterfully over the years.

Yet I was not wholly ignorant of the cumulative effects of such absentee parenthood on children. I had watched business associates suffer morosely through divorces, family counseling, juvenile court appearances, and teen-age drugs.

"Can't understand the boy. Gave the little sonofabitch everything. Now look what he's gone and done to his mother and me. What the hell's wrong with kids today? Why, if I'd ever tried a stunt like that, my old man would have kicked my ass all over main street."

Exactly. Which was probably the reason he never got into any serious trouble. Father fear. Swift punishment. No tolerance of excuses. The way my dad treated me. It might not have been Solomonic wisdom but it worked. It worked because fathers took time to talk to sons and daughters, regarding them gravely as people, not perpetual domiciled annoyances to be tolerated between global business trips or television station breaks. If it had been planned we couldn't have discovered a swifter method of destroying our children or alienating us from their affection.

A few wise among us offer occasional reminders through a form of Madison Avenue consciousness: "Do you know where your child is tonight?" "Be a Big Brother" or "Big Sister." "When was the last time you hugged your kid?" There are camps, foster homes, day-care centers, an entire sociological fabric created out of parental indifference. Parents who are too busy, too tired, too bored, too selfish, or too drunk to care. A heart attack can bring it all into perspective.

"Dad?"

"Uhhuh."

"I've been wondering. When this is all over, I mean when you get better and they release you, will we still be rich like we used to be?"

"You mean money rich?"

Because money no longer seems that important to me. It can never buy health or a replacement for that 10 percent of my heart.

"Not exactly," he says thoughtfully. "But I guess we'd have to have money to afford the things that matter."

"Do we?"

I'm being obtuse, but I want to hear him talk.

"Sure, you know, like living in a big house again and having a heated swimming pool and two cars and a riding lawnmower and being able to go to fun places and eat out at neat restaurants on weekends. That sort of thing."

"We may have to scale our expectations down a little for a while."

"Does that mean we're broke?"

"It does."

"But how come?" He puts down his cards, three short of gin. "I mean, if you really were guilty of stealing millions, why aren't we rich? How come there's nothing left? How come Mum's on welfare? Why didn't you get the best lawyers to defend you instead of defending yourself? How come we went from the top of the world to the bottom? I don't understand!"

His clear brown eyes fill with angry tears. Four years of frustration bubble to the surface of his emotions. He remembers standing on the mountain, seeing me climbing toward the peak. Now we're all in the canyon struggling for survival. No longer can he anticipate his future after seeing the destruction of his past. We have never spoken about such matters man to man. To him the reasons remain shrouded in mystery. Only the results of our destruction are visible: the house in London in which he spent the first ten years of life is gone forever, along with his friends, his climbing tree, his secret hiding places, his memories. Even his bedroom furniture was sold at public auction to provide the money necessary to pay bills and eat.

He remembers the phalanx of policemen armed with search warrants storming through the house—his home— seizing "evidence" while pawing through his toys, his sister's bedrooms, looking for heaven knows what. He remembers the two trials that lasted six months and took four years to conclude.

Three weeks ago he visited me in prison and I congratulated him proudly for doing so well on his Christmas exams. The cons put on a party for the children, Santa Claus arrived, and for a while happiness came peeping from under misery's gray blanket for an hour or more. Now he sees me in hospital and wonders if the story of my recovery is bravado to ease his acceptance of yet another loss. He wants the truth. But sometimes truth is hard to find, let alone tell. . . .

Van Nuys, California

23 April 1975

On the east side of Van Nuys Airport is a complex of hangars and offices occupied by American Jet Industries. Outside on the concrete ramps workmen and mechanics swarm over a dozen different heavy aircraft types, modifying, overhauling, servicing. Yawning cargo doors and new heavy-duty flooring are being installed on a group of Lockheed Electras, a gigantic Guppy is sealed for storage, two Boeing 707s are in the process of modification to executive use, a C-130 Hercules is having an engine change. Noise and clatter are everywhere, combined with the lovely smells of hydraulic fluid, zinc chromate, and arc welding. A visit to AJI stirs the imagination of any aviation buff. "What if ...?" The concept is creativity.

The company is operated by Bill Paulson, an unlikely-looking entrepreneur with inquisitive eyes and soft words. In aviation circles his name is a household word, a man of the same caliber as William Lear, designer of the Learjet. Paulson, too, is a pilot, inventor, designer, engineer, and businessman. An affable dreamer who turns novel aviation ideas into reality and confounds the skeptics. One of a dying breed.

I have come to cut a deal for AJI to finish the engineering, licensing, and inspection of several DC-7 aircraft sitting at Midair's base in the Mojave Desert. It is the last step of the financial and development journey that began when Peter Cheeseman visited me at my swimming pool five years and a thousand heartbreaks ago.

In the last few weeks I have obtained a written commitment for six million dollars' financing from Germany in exchange for 51 percent of the company, and made an agreement with a British company to provide all crewing, maintenance, and management of Midair's global spraying operations. Every company and personal debt will be paid. Every investor will share the good fortune. Finally, and best of all, I will be able to curtail the frantic pace at which I have been working for these past years, narrowing my responsibilities to marketing and technical advice. In every business creation the time arrives when the entrepreneur must step aside and allow a professional management team to take over. For Midair that time has arrived.

Before getting down to business, Paulson wants to show me his latest creation. We walk to a small workshop off the main hangar where he pulls a cover from a wood mock-up. It is to be a single-engine turboprop high-altitude aircraft capable of 400-mph-plus speeds. Aimed for the executive market, it has the capability of landing and taking off from virtually any airport in the world. But the biggest selling feature will be its fuel efficiency.

His mock-up looks sleek and fast. I step through the opening into the main cabin. In comfort it will seat six, ten in a pinch. I feel his dream envelop me. "What if . . . ?"

"Fuel costs," he says quietly. "That will be the deciding factor in selling aircraft for the next decade. How far will it go on how little? That will be the question. The day of the gas guzzlers is gone."

We go back to the office to cut our deal for his work on the DC-7 sprayers—each one a 380-gallon-an-hour gas guzzler. Food for thought.

The idea of using four-engine propeller-driven passenger planes as agricultural and forestry sprayers—gigantic crop dusters—was proven practical in 1972.

After our four machines arrived safely in Long Beach from Kenai, Alaska, in late February, a test site was arranged at Daggett Airport near the town of Barstow in the Mojave Desert. Hot, flat, desolate country where sidewinders ridged the parched sandy soil and on rare days the humidity touched 8 percent. Nights were cold and star-bright. We moved one airplane to Daggett Airport so that I could spend a few hours familiarizing myself with this seventy-ton-gross-weight behemoth. Strangely, the DC-7 turned out to be a docile brute, easy to fly with no bad habits. A bit heavy on the controls perhaps at low speeds, but giving lots of advance warning when it didn't like the way it was being handled.

After a few cautious hours aloft, for we were all novices, any apprehension vanished and I had us streaking over the early-morning desert a few feet above the ground at close to 300 mph. Once we felt comfortable and the crew were satisfied that I wouldn't drive us into the side of a hill, the experts from Canada were invited down to evaluate our spraying capabilities.

They arrived during the first week of March, delighted to be escaping winter's northern grip. A federal government research team headed by A. P. Randall brought special equipment for exact measurement of the aircraft's swath width and spray-drop pattern. Quebec forestry officials under Gerrard Paquet were there to crosscheck the findings.

During the week I flew at various altitudes and airspeeds and in a variety of wind conditions in order to establish the best criteria for operation. I had only the vaguest idea of what would happen and had been basing all my theories on utilizing the effects of wake turbulence produced by heavy aircraft to carry the fine spray particles on a horizontal whirlwind farther than had ever been done before.

Imagine a motorboat skimming the ocean at twenty knots. Its wake can be measured in a few feet on either side of the hull before disappearing in a stir of water. But put a two-hundred-thousand-ton tanker on the same ocean at twenty knots and the sheer force of its bulk and displacement will create a sizable wave for a mile on either side of its course. Airborne, the same rules should apply . . . in theory.

The tests were concluded by the end of the week, with much of it recorded on some spectacular film footage. Results proved that the DC-7 could produce an effective swath width of three thousand feet flying at not less than 240 mph and two hundred feet above the ground. This was at least ten times better aircraft performance than anyone had seen used on forestry spraying. The Quebec government kept its word: a million-dollar contract was ours. No official legal documents, meetings with accountants, or other such nonsense, just a precise two-line telegram of confirmation—in English. We were all ecstatic.

The world was ours. By cutting spraying costs by 80 percent and increasing efficiency tenfold, the DC-7 could serve an invaluable need to increase food production throughout the world in those areas where agricultural losses to disease and insects devastated whole nations and their economies. Rice crops in the Far East, sugar cane in Brazil, cotton in the Sudan and Pakistan, wheat in the Ukraine, fruit-fly spraying in Mexico and Central America, tsetse-fly control in Africa, forestry spraying in Scadinavia and North America—the opportunities were legion. We would build the company into a fleet of twenty, perhaps thirty, aircraft with mother ships carrying supplies of spare parts and portable workshops. We could deal in barter with Third World countries that had no hard currency. We would become multimillionaires and grow old and fat and envied and live happily ever after, amen.

Practically, we should have waited another year to perfect the jerry-built system we'd created. It was a plumber's nightmare. Time was needed to work out its shortcomings. Additionally, much more flight testing was required with the Litton INS—Inertial Navigational System—I intended using because I was not at all satisfied that it was going to function on low-level spraying operations exactly the way Litton Industries claimed.

But we didn't have the money to survive another year of tests and experiments. Besides, the Quebec forestry people believed now in our ability to perform. After all, they had seen the aircraft operate successfully during its week of trials.

They were on the ground. I was in the cockpit. From the cockpit nothing worked properly. The shut-off valves leaked. No problem when the liquid is a stove-oil and red-dye mixture, but absolutely lethal to everyone on board if the liquid is a highly volatile insecticide. On each of our twenty-second runs across the desert check area the electric motor driving the spray pump overheated alarmingly. What would happen under actual working conditions when it had to run continuously for twenty minutes or more? I was afraid to try and find out until the government observers left. The aircraft's number-three engine refused to deliver full power at take-off. No problem while we were flying with a five-hundred-gallon spray load under ideal conditions, but what would happen taking off from a short bush strip with five thousand gallons on board? And as if all this wasn't enough to curl my hair, every one of our newly installed internal tanks so carefully anchored to the floor of the central cabin worked themselves loose from their moorings during normal airborne vibrations. I shuddered to think what might happen in rough air with full spray tanks.

Clearly, we needed time to regroup, replace, and repair. For the moment we were a low-level disaster remaining aloft through a mixture of luck and prayer.

When the tests ended, I took the DC-7 back to Long Beach with a long repair list for Cheeseman and his mechanics. He promised to have it ready in time for the spraying season. A second machine I flew through to Toronto in mid-March. There were no DC-7 aircraft licensed or operating in Canada; therefore replacement parts or major components needed during our spray operations would have to be provided by us. The Toronto-based machine could be cannibalized as required. With luck it wouldn't be necessary.

Once word of Quebec's intentions was known around Canadian aviation circles, a great lament arose about how Midair's aircraft would be taking business away from the smaller, less efficient machines used for so long on the Canadian forestry programs in Quebec and on the East Coast. If one big plane could do the work of fifteen smaller ones, then fifteen pilots, aircraft, and mechanics would be unemployed. Representations were made to the federal government to prevent the aircraft from entering Canada. Fortunately, Quebec's political lobby and Francophone stubbornness prevailed and on the twenty-fourth of May I landed at Lac des Loups in northern Quebec to begin operations with our repaired and rejuvenated monster.

It still wasn't working properly. The Litton INS, tied into the aircraft's autopilot, took us on all sorts of strange airborne meanderings contrary to the guarantees of its programming experts, and the spray motor still overheated. But we had run out of time. The spruce budworm had hatched and was feeding on the trees. We took out the first 5,000-gallon load two days later, lumbering into the air at dawn with our fingers crossed.

As in the Mojave, our spray blocks were scattered with check cards to assess the droplet pattern in effective spray coverage. By the second day we were managing a one-hour turnaround time and completing 25,000 acres a load. Everything went wrong. The tanks leaked, the motors on the pump kept burning out, the valves stuck open—or closed—the INS was useless, and two cylinders cracked on the aircraft's number-three engine. But we stuck it out and fought it through.

Work hours began at dawn and ended during late morning when the ground warmed, sending the light spray particles aloft. Evening hours began when the air cooled and winds died and usually gave us no more than a couple of hours' working time. It was just as well. Every precious minute of ground time was needed to make the discreet repairs necessary in order to be ready for the next spray period. For the mechanics it was a nightmare of overwork—day and night—under primitive conditions and fighting the fury of black flies that swarmed in cyclones as the sun went down.

I had leased a twin-engine courier aircraft to race for spare parts in Ottawa or Toronto as we needed them. It seemed to be in the air day and night. Everything we had brought with us on the spares inventory turned out to be things we didn't need because they didn't—or wouldn't—break down. At one point a young mechanic was dispatched by airplane to Los Angeles for more electric pump motors. He traveled without sleep for two days and nights, bringing them back as excess baggage for a total ticket cost that could have taken any one of us around the world first class with enough left over for a Caribbean cruise. We had to succeed. The national daily papers, CBC News, foreign visitors from Japan, the United States and the Scandinavian countries kept dropping by to watch and question.

After a week, when I was certain that we could finish the work and keep the aircraft aloft, I phoned Larry Mudgett in California, the ex-Pan Am captain who had checked me out on the DC-7 initially, and asked if he would fly up to Canada and take over so that I could go back to the job of raising funds needed for the next stage of Midair's development. He arrived on the courier aircraft the next afternoon in time for the evening spray period. I packed my bags and wished him luck.

As every businessman knows, a new company based on a concept or a novel idea requiring unknown amounts of technical research before being perfected for market is nearly impossible to finance through conventional lending institutions. By definition, banks and trust companies are skeptical and chary of the untried or novel innovation. Despite their advertising to the contrary, I have yet to meet a bank or lending institution willing to lend or invest in a situation involving R and D, entrepreneurial development, or pursuit of a new market of opportunity. I cannot blame them. Their loans are made against some form of tangible security that, in the event of business failure, can be resold to cover their client's indebtedness. Vintage passenger airliners with guts removed and smelly spray tanks installed don't fit that category.

So, what are termed euphemistically as "oddball" lenders must be found, risk takers who are prepared to invest a little—or a lot—in hopes of getting a hell of a lot more in return. Without them, new ideas wither on the vine of dreams and eventually die.

Like all life on earth, a new company begins with sperm capital, cash from the progenitor's pockets used to pay legal fees for company formation, print the first business cards and office stationery, buy second-hand furniture, pay the rent and the telephone.

Seed capital is the next rung on the growth ladder, where banks, family, and relations are tapped on a personally secured basis to provide the funds required to continue functioning until the first revenues are assured and a cash flow established. With Midair's Quebec contract for one DC-7, plus the usual summer spray work for the firm's single-engine aircraft, we were ready for the next financial step: venture capital.

Venture capital is brave money from professional risk takers who invest on the basis of company management, soundness of the idea presented, how much money the principals have poured into the business so far, and of course the long-term rewards. In exchange for their bravery they demand high interest and a good slice of company stock. Not at all unreasonable.

Eric Schwendau and I began beating the bushes for money. He went after professional private lenders while I went after the federal government in Ottawa. The Department of Trade and Industry indicated a willingness to assist with grant money in order to help us develop the sprayers for the export market. A variety of funding sources for grant monies were available under trick titles and acronyms: PAIT, IRDIA, DREE, and so forth. Over the months and years that followed my initial overtures, Trade and Industry were most helpful in paving the way with introductions through our embassies to various interested government officials and prospects from the private sector in many different countries, but never once did I see a cent of financial assistance in spite of several applications and verbal promises.

Yet they did steer me to a contact in Egypt that I thought worth further investigation. A request for technical assistance had been received from Cairo, explaining Egypt's need for spray planes to control seasonal insects on their huge cotton acreage. Czech and Polish crop-dusting firms were doing the work under bilateral trade agreements arranged through Russia. But with Nasser's death and Sadat's growing unease about Egypt's army of Russian "advisers," the decision had been made to look for help in the West. Would I be interested in going to Egypt for an on-site assessment of their situation? You bet I would.

After making hurried arrangements for short-term financing to carry company operations through the rest of the summer, and a quick trip to Halifax to visit Helen and the children for my birthday party at her parents' home where they spent each summer, Eric and I left for Europe and the Middle East.

Although Midair was our principal interest, we had a number of other irons in the development fire, any one of which would make us instant multimillionaires if brought to fruition. These included a line of plastic beer bottles developed by a genial Swiss engineer that was going to stop the breweries from burying the country in cans; a sale of fighter aircraft from Venezuela's air force to Pakistan for their next war with India; a humidity machine company—called Humidex, what else?— with a product developed for hospitals to maintain perfect moisture control for patients under anesthetic during long operations; emeralds from Colombia—bought from real mountain bandits—to sell for cutting in Brussels and Israel; industrial diamonds and gold bullion from Brazil; a new record-company promotion for the Christmas season; plus a host of other ideas and ventures that kept coming to us every week from would-be entrepreneurs and dreamers. Some were excellent; most, completely nuts. We studied them all, fascinated by the combination of genius and lunacy that swarmed on all sides. Now that Midair had apparently taken off against impossible odds, word was out that we were winners with money to spend and a magic touch for success. How little they knew.

First stop was England for discussions with Vickers Manufacturing in Basingstoke on the humidity machines, then on to The Hague for talks with WHO—World Health Organization—about their planned large-scale spraying in Upper Volta to control an insect that caused river blindness to the area's inhabitants. Next, we flew north to Copenhagen and Oslo, advertising our wares to the Scandinavian countries that had expressed interest in using the DC-7 on forestry insects in their nations. In Prague we had a weapons conference with directors from the Skoda Works: arms and munitions were needed for Pakistan. Could they deliver in time? They would let us know. On to Zurich for the Swiss beer bottler and his brown plastic jugs, which he threatened would one day roll around the world. Milan, Rome, Teheran, Kuwait, and a bewildering round of meetings, conferences, hearty handshakes, deceitful winks, and delightful anecdotes. Everyone with an angle to make a fortune or with a fortune to spend on a good angle. Finally we arrived in Cairo on Japan Airlines at two in the morning.

Egypt was not a place to visit in August. It sat stifling under a mantle of heat and cloudless dun-colored sky. The new Hilton Hotel was filled with squat, smelly Russians in heavy serge suits and wilting ties: humorless-looking men with peasant faces and steel teeth. They didn't appear to like anything or anyone, themselves included, and after squeezing in next to several in a cramped elevator I could understand why. Deodorants could develop into a definite growth industry behind the Iron Curtain, should anyone care to pursue the matter.

Once a pearl of cities on par with Paris or London, Cairo had not worn well under Nasser. In the process of making social progress a uniform mediocrity had been achieved to the extent that nothing—from telephones, taps, and toilets to transport, trains, and taxis—worked properly. Government offices bulged with clerks carrying rubber stamps—sharing one ink pad—whose sole function appeared to be adding stamps to reams of already-stamped papers, then passing them along for someone else to stamp. Employment creativity with a very small "e." Shops and windows along the main streets had been boarded up, their entrances hidden behind massive sandbags.

"You're expecting trouble?" I inquired of Aziz Ezzat, our new Egyptian agent.

"Israelis," he explained. "They come over in their fighters at low level, breaking the sound barrier and all the windows. Then they sweep up to Alexandria on the way home and do the same thing there. Bastards!"

"Why don't your shoot them down?"

"With what?"

"Missiles and airplanes. You have MIGs and SAMs. Use them."

He gave a sour, derisive laugh at my naïveté. "Our air force is grounded because the Russians won't send us any tires. Five landings and a MIG needs new tires. No tires, no operational aircraft. The army won't trust anyone with the SAMs since our glorious soldiers kept shooting down the Illuyshin passenger aircraft flying between Cairo and Alexandria. Now we have no SAMs, and if you want to get to Alexandria it is necessary to drive or take the train."

"You are joking."

"Air Marshal Bogdady is a good friend. I know many things that aren't for publication. This country is the joke."

Understandably he was bitter. His family owned large estates before Nasser. He went to England for his education, graduating from Cambridge with an engineering degree and a love of flying. After World War II he joined Egyptair, flying old De Havilland Dragon Rapides across the Middle East. When Nasser came to power everything Ezzat had was swept away in the resulting frenzy of nationalism and equality for the masses. Now Sadat had invited the exiles home to repair the economy and the nation. There were promises of full restitution for what was seized, either in kind or in cash. Was it a mirage? Time would tell. Under a hot August sun everything moves slowly in the Middle East.

He took us to the Ministry of Agriculture for meetings with the minister and his deputies. Everyone spoke English, French, and Arabic, three-sided conversations in three languages ensued. Arabic for noncommittal comment, French for polite political inquiry and good manners, English for specifics and a thrust of words from behind which it is impossible to hide.

Yes, we had permission to travel north to visit the cotton areas and to leave the main roads to examine the fields and talk to growers. A permit would be arranged at once. Could our big planes carry Egyptian fruit and vegetables to Europe? There was a need to develop hard-currency markets quickly. The East Block countries had been taking everything for credits, but what good were credits when there was no money for the farmer?

The minister had a point. Ezzat jumped in with a burst of Arabic and the minister nodded his understanding. I felt uneasy at these Arabic exchanges of which I was not a part. Were we committing our resources unwittingly?

A servant appeared carrying a brass filigree tray covered with tiny coffee cups. He moved slowly around the room in an obsequious shuffle, ignored by the Egyptians. Both Eric and I thanked the man in French. He gave a startled smile and nearly dropped the tray. Ezzat looked annoyed, the others puzzled.

From the high and very dirty ceiling a quartet of enormous wooden paddles stirred the leaden air in a desultory fashion, producing neither breeze nor relief within the dust-choked room. We showed our color film of the DC-7 operating in Canada and the United States. The Egyptians liked the show. Movies in the morning with their coffee. Just the thing to start the day.

The road to Alexandria was a narrow, crowded thorough-fare filled with beggars, potholes, and swaying camels, the latter staring haughtily at Ezzat's white air-conditioned Chevrolet Impala as we horned our way through the throngs of burdened beasts. We crossed endless canals and waterways, all part of the Nile and its intricate irrigation networks that spider up from Cairo in a huge triangle flooding the Delta. Heat and humidity on the Delta were quite different from the city, a soggy oppressiveness.

After an hour we turned off on a side road—hard-packed earth and sand that looked and felt like tanned concrete. The farms were so small. Irregular-shaped fields were cluttered with date palms and towering eucalyptus, each farm edged by crumbling adobe-style houses with mud patty-pie walls, dung fire, and filthy children scrabbling in the dirt. Blindfolded oxen walked in lethargic circles on the end of a pole connected to a primitive water wheel. Brown liquid splashed along slipways to the crops. Fellahin dressed in gray skullcaps and striped nightshirts glanced at us indifferently. Their poverty crushed against the senses. The cradle of civilization. In five thousand years nothing had changed. Nor was it likely to change over the next five millennia. We pulled off the road to park and climbed out. Heat hit us like a mallet.

"Ask him if he is getting good insect control."

Ezzat blasted the poor farmer with Arabic. Hearing anyone speak this language, one has the impression that an argument is raging, violence ready to explode. Not so. It is the manner of the idiom, guttural sounds similar to Turkish or German. Courting a woman in Arabic, to Western ears, is like an overture to rape.

The farmer, a stunted old-young man with burnished mahogany features and thick, powerful hands that built the world, explained shyly how the spray pilots were stealing his insecticides because he was a poor man. He was unable to afford the baksheesh necessary for a first-class job. Once he complained to a local government man who turned out to be working with the pilots. All he got for his efforts was a beating from the police for trying to make trouble for the distinguished foreign guests. He finished with a resigned, nearly toothless smile and shrugged.

"It is the Will of Allah," Ezzat translated. "The man is a goddamn fool. Let's go."

We remained in Egypt for ten days, seeing the sights, crawling through traffic to business meetings with incredulous government officials, crawling through mosques, temples, museums, pyramids, and night life at "Tent City" in the Cairo outskirts of El Giza. Crawling into bed.

Finally, armed with assurances that our bid to spray the country's cotton on a three-year contract using fifty small aircraft would be received favorably by the new Sadat government if we cared to submit our tender, we left for Athens.

Democracy's cradle had been suffering from totalitarianism.

The Greek military dictatorship had ended. The colonels were in prison and the government was anxious to turn every commercial enterprise they had operated back to the private sector from which it had been seized. This included the annual spraying operations for malaria, cotton, and olives throughout the Hellenic Isles.

A strange little brigadier (Ret.) sporting an eye patch and a limp conducted us through a series of conferences and clandestine meetings with military officers while we tried to sort out exactly what it was that they wanted. Under the colonels, everything had been conducted so secretly for so long that subterfuge had become a way of life. Our problem was the drachma's convertibility into hard currency to purchase chemicals for their various programs. The government wanted to pay in drachma instead of produce, insisting that we pay all wages and local purchases in American dollars.

"But what do we do with all the drachma if it can't be taken out of the country or converted into dollars?" Eric demanded at one of our surreptitious meetings.

"Build hotels!" the brigadier (Ret.) suggested brightly. "Greece always needs more tourist hotels. And I, George Demetrius Papadopolos, will be happy to assist in your new hotel operations."

Beware of limping Greeks with eye patches.

Back to Canada in time for the Labor Day weekend. The season was over, except for four small aircraft sent to Nicaragua for the cotton spraying there. The difference between revenues and expenditures was frightening. We needed a corporate angel to take us on board. The world might have been at our feet but the creditors and shareholders were on our backs demanding faster action, progress, new contracts. Money.

I tried Brascan, the Canadian-Brazilian giant of Bay Street and Rio de Janeiro. Its chairman, Jake Moore, was intrigued by the possibilities of global agricultural-spray operations. He turned me over to a team of economic analysts and lizard-lipped accountants to work out five-year projections on Midair's anticipated earnings. Star-gazing in the grand sense. Unpaid and under pressure to put the mirage and marriage together, I worked like a demon for weeks.

Brascan didn't like Eric Scwendau as president. A personal matter. Eric and I discussed the situation and decided to trade titles. I became president. What's in a name? Brascan wanted all Midair's shares collected and signed over from the existing shareholders for full payout on the day of merger. We raced off to get them. The weeks passed. October. November. Ezzat phoned from Beirut—impossible to make a call out of Egypt because the connections were so bad—he wanted to know what had happened to our nine-million-dollar bid on the Egyptian spraying? Cairo was waiting to sack the Poles and Czechs. Brascan stalled, they demanded payment in gold. Cairo agreed. A courier was dispatched to the Middle East with our tender and deposit money.

Two weeks later we were notified that the contract was ours. Brascan was forced to a commitment. Greed took over. Their directors decided to change our original agreement. Frank Lewarren, vice president of industrial development, hit me at the Brascan employee Christmas party: "Now this fifty-five percent equity for Brascan and forty-five for your people just won't wash, Tony."

"Oh?"

He held my arm confidentially, guiding me to a vacant wall space out of earshot from the milling revelers.

"Now that everything is coming into focus, Jake feels that our initial understanding should be based more on the present realities than on wishful thinking. I agree. What do you think?"

"I think we had a deal. Fifty-five, forty-five."

"You're not being realistic. Midair's broke. Without us you're finished. You're worried about your own position? Don't be. There's a spot for you on our home team. Stock options, the works. Jake likes you. Ted Freeman-Atwood likes you. I like you too."

"I'm flattered. But the deal is still fifty-five, forty-five."

"Not any more it isn't." His face hardened, along with the grip on my elbow. "We've decided on eighty-five percent for Brascan, fifteen for the Midair group. What do you say to that?"

"I say, go fuck yourself, Frank."

Brave, stupid words, which accomplished nothing except personal satisfaction. Merry Christmas 1972. Four months of hard work down the drain for nothing.

In Egypt the Poles and Czechs won our three-year contract by default. In Nicaragua there was an earthquake and our local partner and manager, Armando Rivas, disappeared together with his wife and children under the rubble that once had been the city of Managua. We lost four aircraft, all our parts supply, company records, and any hope of collecting monies due from customers. Most of them were wiped out too. Within the week word of Brascan's split had reached the ears of Quebec's forestry people and we were notified diplomatically that our DC-7 would not be welcome on the 1973 spray program. Later we discovered that Conair of Abbottsford, B.C.—the company that shared the Lac des Loups airfield with Midair and whose engineers had photographed every portion of our DC-7's spray system—had converted two DC-6 aircraft and were leasing additional four-engined machines from the United States to work in Quebec. They did not want to see us on the job. I was speechless with anger.

The year 1973 had to be better. Impossible to believe a new year worse than 1972. Nor, as things turned out, was it. Eric, who had anticipated a Brascan about-face after they insisted on his removal as Midair's president, had been out scouring the Toronto financial community for a likely angel. He uncovered exactly what was needed in D. Gordon Badger—complete with white suit, wings, and slightly tarnished halo. Just our sort of angel.

Badger, a bright, personable six-footer with prematurely gray curly hair, had been responsible for the development and huge success of *Homemaker's Digest*. A Clarkson-and-Gordon-trained accountant, he'd created Holdex Group, a company designed for developing or factoring "Deals" on behalf of a coterie of high-flying investors with tax problems: lawyers, doctors, businessmen, real estate millionaires, and accountants like himself.

He dealt in the improbable world of numbers and projections. Navel-gazing in the abstract. But he liked Midair's—really Brascan's—five-year projections and decided with little preamble to back us for a third of the action. Our attorneys drew up the papers and Midair married Badger and his Holdex Group.

By early spring over a million dollars of new financing appeared. Debts were paid. Employees hired. A fleet of surplus DC-7 aircraft purchased for conversion. An operational base opened and staffed under Peter Cheeseman's direction at

Daggett Airport in California. An international business consultant and former chief executive officer of Salada-Shirrif-Horsey
contracted to develop foreign markets. Head office moved into
the Holdex building on University Avenue in downtown
Toronto, and I began putting in some incredibly long working
hours sandwiched in between global sales trips. Heady times. I
ate junk food, lost weight, and developed a nervous tic.

To avoid the commuting problem, I took a bachelor
apartment in downtown Toronto and drove home on weekends
to London to see Helen and the children. Generally I was too
tired to spend much time with them, or too busy working on the
bulging files I'd brought along. I smoked like a chimney, became
short-tempered, irritable with delays, racing to meet one
deadline after another and never satisfied with my performance.
There was always a crisis somewhere that needed instant
attention and solution. Nervous bankers, wary creditors needing
encouragement, balking suppliers, anxious shareholders.

Original estimates for certifying each DC-7 in the United
States to FAA standards as rebuilt aircraft had been set by
Cheeseman at a quarter of a million dollars. It was difficult to
argue with the chief engineer and a principal shareholder over
his figures. The first six machines would be airborne and ready
for work by October 1973, then one every four months
thereafter until our fleet was at full operational strength by the
end of the following year. No problem.

On paper it sounded wonderful and Badger seemed happy
with the figures, but I should have been alert enough to hire a
second opinion instead of relying wholly on Yorkshire-style
optimism. To be on the safe side I added 50 percent to the
budget for cost overruns and put down December as the earliest
date for our first aircraft delivery. Cheeseman moved his family
to Barstow and bought a home. He loved the desert life and the
grandeur of running his own show with only a single umbilical
Telex line connecting him to Head Office in Toronto. Not since
World War II had Daggett Airport seen such aviation activity.

With production targets settled and sufficient funding
arranged for the year, I turned next to the problem of markets

for our big birds. In Rome, FAO—the Food and Agriculture Organization branch of the United Nations—guided me to those countries they considered to be most receptive and in need of what Midair had to offer. I drew up a list of places to visit: Pakistan, India, South Africa, Malaysia, Indonesia, Libya, Egypt, Iran, Colombia, Trinidad, Panama, France, Germany—the list went on and on.

I traveled with one or more of our technical consultants and visited the world. An FAO contract was obtained in Africa for aerial seeding of the drought-stricken Sahel in Upper Volta, a stand-by contract was offered by the Desert Locust Control Commission for an aircraft to be based in Saudi Arabia. Malaria spraying was under negotiation in both Venezuela and Brazil, the latter wanting the entire Amazon Highway cleared of infection. Nigeria wanted a multimillion-dollar job done near Kaduna for control of the tsetse fly. Pakistan wanted two DC-7s to spray the valley of the Indus for cotton and citrus insects. Cyprus needed Mediterranean fruit-fly control over the entire island. A hundred million dollars' worth of business was ours for the taking.

But when December came and I flew out to California, Midair had run out of money, material, and credit. The two DC-7s on the production line appeared no closer to FAA certification than in the spring. Because someone in a fit of false economy had refused to pay a niggardly storage bill for a few thousand dollars at the Sebring, Florida, airport, six of our newly purchased aircraft were seized, together with parts and spares, and quickly sold at a neatly contrived sheriff's sale. All quite legal, although hardly above board. Total losses came to nearly two hundred thousand dollars—a blow from which the company never fully recovered. I was furious.

New budget revisions now came to $750,000 per aircraft, with the first promised absolutely, positively, for May 1974. So much had been spent on FAA certification that it seemed foolish to cancel the program at that point and revert to flying under the "experimental" category. Now, in retrospect, it seems that that is what should have been done.

By the following summer, when certification still had not been completed and all of our various in-house get-rich-quick schemes foundered, Midair began to come apart, bringing with it Badger and Holdex. Sheriff's notices appeared on our office doors.

By the end of the year Cheeseman had joined a new company based at Daggett and shrugged off the Midair fiasco as no further concern of his. He bought himself a new and bigger home in Apple Valley near cowboy star Roy Rogers and did very well for himself.

Eric Schwendau, after losing everything he owned—which had been considerable—lost his wife in a messy divorce and opened a small consulting company in Toronto's Cabbagetown which was just on the verge of clicking for him when misfortune once again came charging from the sidelines.

All Midair's employee's and consultants departed until I was left in a single crumbling room in an old house on Wellesley Street surrounded by filing cabinets, flaking woodwork, and fragmented dreams. To say that 1974 ended on a low point would be an understatement. Yet in three months with a burst of frantic energy I managed to put most of the corporate wreckage back together again in such a manner that full recovery was possible for everyone of us, including Cheeseman.

American Jet Industries at Van Nuys and Bill Paulson are my keystone. AJI will finish certification of the DC-7s, Mike Keegan's British Air Ferries in Southend, England, will operate them, and the German group from Frankfurt will pay out all debts for 51 percent of the company, giving every shareholder three dollars for each dollar invested. The journey is over.

I sit in Paulson's office with Keegan waiting for Bill Bone, AJI's chief planner, to arrive. The room is big and easy, like the man who lives in it. Scatterings of photographs and plaques adorn the walls; table mementos have been shoved aside to make way for engineering reports and drawings. Chaos and orderliness are everywhere. For the first time in years I feel completely relaxed, filled with that confidence which comes with the knowledge of success. A good feeling.

The desk phone rings. Paulson picks it up.

"It's for you. Long distance."

I lean on the edge of his desk. Outside, a propjet screams in reverse pitch. Dust lifts against the window in fine flecks.

"Tony?"

It's my brother calling from Toronto.

"We've got trouble here." His voice is tremulous. "The police have just raided the office and taken everything—files, books, typewriters, everything. They cleaned Eric's office out as well. His house. My house. Your house. Ten or fifteen locations on the search warrants. You'd better come home."

A pain knifes against my breast. I struggle for air. There is none. My telephone arm goes numb for a moment. Dark waves and dancing lights leap about the room. Then everything comes back into focus—sounds, sights, smells. The others are talking. Bill Bone has arrived and is being introduced. In my heart I know it is the end. One journey is over. Another is about to begin. . . .

Kingston, Canada

24 January 1980

Mr. Leader died last night. It happened after midnight. Hoarse shouts for help: he couldn't breathe. Those strong fingers that had shaped a thousand monuments into velvet granite tore frantically at his arrested heart, then were stilled forever.

Doctors and nurses came running. A resuscitator careened against the door in a clatter of castering wheels and oxygen bottles. It was a replay of the previous week when I was under surveillence in the fishbowl and the old woman had given up and died.

They raced their lifesaving machines and drugs and knowledge into Mr. Leader's room and fought for his life. They pounded and shouted and cursed. But it was no use. Mr. Leader's gentle spirit had fled.

I didn't get out of bed to investigate. There was no need. Mr. Sung looked across the dim space that separated our beds and nodded gravely. Mr. Sung and I, two shipwrecked sailors on our solitary island surrounded by shark-infested waters. We listened to the frantic forces trying valiantly to beat back the sharks on that island next door. After a time, silence descended and Mr. Leader's slack-jawed corpse went wheeling past our door on its way to eternity.

Unlike that immediacy of death in war, traffic accidents, or aviation disasters, hospital death touches the very marrow of our being. It is not a matter of chance, such as an exploding mortar hurling us into slivers of meat and bone, or a stray bullet drilling a neat brown hole in the middle of our forehead, a tractor-trailer jackknifing on the highway before our eyes and flipping twenty tons of cargo in an instant to squash us flat, or an exploding airliner turning everyone on board into screaming, thick strawberry jam as it hits the ground seven miles below at

104

the speed of sound. These things always happen to the other fellow. Never us. Perhaps because it happens so quickly, there isn't time to reflect. One is either participant or observer with everything clearly defined.

In hospitals it is quite different. Without exception, we are all participants, viewing divergent paths of our mortality. No choices are given. Some Greater Power in the natural order of things will decide. No one wants to know the exact method, day, and hour anyway. It would spoil the game for all of us.

But did Mr. Leader know? When I talked to him he acted like a man vouchsafed more than a glimpse of what lay beyond. I wonder. Perhaps just before each journey some curtain in the subconscious parts and there is a vision of gliding over the waters to eternal peace. It is comforting to think so. Meanwhile my curtain remains firmly closed and life proceeds.

The eleventh day dawns bright and clear and very cold. Hoarfrost clutches the trees, wires, and cartops. Smoke plumes from bundled pedestrians; vehicle exhausts wreathe the streets and sidewalks below my window. A few puffy sparrows search for morsels along the salted gutters.

I breakfast, bathe, shave, and lie waiting for doctor's rounds. Finally, near ten, Dr. Koval arrives with entourage, an emperor in white who has somehow managed to retain the common touch. Does he realize the effect that his presence produces on patients? He must. He takes my pulse, listens to my chest pumping serenely, and smiles.

"You can check out this morning. I'll leave a prescription order at the nurses' desk. Pick it up when you go."

"A prescription? For what?"

"Digoxin—that's a trade name for digitalis."

I remember reading an Ellery Queen mystery in which the murderer gave an overdose of the foxglove derivative to do the foul deed so that he could reap his reward of the victim's estate and beautiful wife. Does anyone read Ellery Queen mysteries nowadays or are they outdated like Nero Wolfe? But there is no parallel in my case: my estate is valueless and Helen far too wise to be trapped by some local Lothario into murdering me. I'm quite safe. But why do I need Digoxin?

"There's a slight irregularity to your heart rhythm. This will provide a little stimulus until it settles back to normal."

The others nod approvingly at his decision. In the face of such overwhelming approbation, who am I to argue the merits of digitalis?

"Anything else I need to take?"

"Yes. For the next six weeks take it easy. Work up to your former level of activity gradually. Don't overdo it. Go slowly. Very slowly on stairs, lots of pauses to rest. Then short walks, and don't lift anything heavy. In two months you should be back to where you were before the attack. Hopefully, you'll never have another problem. Good luck."

Grinning like an idiot, I shake his hand. Remission. The mighty Lord Koval has given his guarantee that I will return to normal. What more do I need? No special diet. No necessity to curtail my activities or work habits. The whole experience has not been a disaster after all, merely a warning that I am into middle age and must expect the machinery to slow down a little. I have been wallowing in a sea of self-pity for nothing. Such a fool.

"You go?" Mr. Sung inquires.

"Damn right. I go!"

I phone Helen with the news. Relief. We laugh. She promises never to use digitalis on me. Mr. Sung watches, nodding and smiling at my good fortune, sharing my delight to be leaving. I wish it were possible to go home to Helen so that we could talk and touch and share. But I can't. It is forbidden. I must return to the place whence I came: I am a convict on parole. Now I call my jailers with the news.

The prison's duty officer tells me curtly there will be a vehicle at the hospital's side door to take me back at eleven-thirty. Return to reality. Such silliness. It would be just as easy to order a taxi or have Helen drive me. But prison bureaucracy prefers doing things its way according to the knee-jerk procedure for inmates—no one is a convict or prisoner these days—on medical leave of absence.

In December, after the first hair-raising ambulance ride to

hospital when I was pronounced fit and released, Helen took me back in her car. Not proper procedure at all. The prison staff were furious. I might have taken it into my head to escape.

"But I didn't. I'm here. See! It's *me*, in the flesh."

"That's not the point. When you do something like this it makes us look bad," the duty officer complained bitterly.

The point was, I discovered later, that there would have been fewer questions asked, fewer problems created, if I had escaped. Simply driven across the border on the Thousand Islands Bridge and vanished into the bowels of the American subsociety along with the other twenty million illegal aliens who live there. But I didn't. Therefore I wasn't playing the game. Papers had to be filled in, explanations made, work created—always an annoyance within the regimen of any bureaucratic system.

It is time to leave. I collect my things, give Mr. Sung a formal bedside bow, wishing him long life, fast recovery, and much happiness. His wife arrives with her shopping bag and newspapers. Seeing me dressed and combed, she chirps a few words.

"Mrs. Sung say you not to come back this place," her husband translates.

"You tell Mrs. Sung that I will do my best to obey her wishes."

When I kiss her smooth cheek she giggles like a teenager. My prescriptions are at the nurses' station: Inderal, Anturan, and Digoxin. The first to hold down my blood pressure and heartbeat, the second to prevent sudden clotting, the third to steady the rhythm.

None of the nurses or interns says good-by. "Good luck!" is their form of adieu. Do they know something I don't? The buxom head nurse reminds me once more to take it easy for the next few weeks, not to do anything silly. Such as what? But she refuses to answer with more than a wink. I have the feeling that none of them expects to see me make it to the lobby, let alone off the premises.

"And don't lift anything heavy."

She glares accusingly at my small overnight bag as if I have broken this rule already. It must weight all of four pounds. An elevator takes me to the main floor and I walk slowly along the corridors to the side entrance. It is an effort. My legs are wobbly, my heart racing. Fortunately there are chairs along the route for intermediate resting. Thoughtful administration.

In the lobby I sit checking my pulse. Fifty-six beats a minute. Normally it used to run between eighty and ninety when walking. Now it doesn't seem to matter whether I walk, sit, or lie down. Fifty-six beats a minute is all I'm going to get. Is this good or bad? I should have asked someone.

Some months later I discover why I am on Digoxin. Heart attack victims who survive the initial attack still face the risk of sudden arrhythmia. For a six-month period after an attack the situation remains critical and 10 percent of the victims succumb to an abnormal heart rhythm. Is it wrong to hold this information from patients? I don't know. Looking back, I can't see that it makes any difference, but perhaps some people tend to worry more than others.

Outside the window across the street, a lake-blue twelve-passenger van pulls to the curb and stops. Its door is lettered in red: SOLICITOR GENERAL. My jailers have come to collect me. My chauffer is a spare saturnine man with gray brush cut and gravel voice who regards the world through a pair of suspicious eyes. I climb in beside him.

"You all right now?" he grates.

"Fine, thanks."

He's trying to be pleasant; I can feel his sympathy reaching out. That unspoken bond which welds all men together in the face of a common adversary. His name is Earl and he is nearing retirement age; the dangerous years, when heart attacks and cancer run roughshod and indiscriminately. Disease is an equal-opportunity employer. A great leveler.

When the Kingston Penitentiary riots of 1971 were quelled and the most dangerous convicts moved to a new maximum-security prison at Millhaven, a jailers' gauntlet was set up to greet them. Forced to run between two lines of club-wielding guards, the men were beaten—some seriously. A subsequent Parliamentary Committee investigating the riot produced over sixty recommendations for improving the system and prison conditions generally, among them that the half-dozen officers involved in that Millhaven incident be transferred to positions within the penitentiary service where they could have no further contact with prisoners. Earl was one of those half-dozen. He and three others from the group were moved to a minumum-security farm camp, exchanging uniforms for mufti and the lesser responsibility—and perhaps temptation—of overseeing the least violent of convicts within the system.

I pity the man. Oddly, I have come to pity all my jailers. Behind their gruff facades, harsh words, and sarcasms, they have turned out to be mere mortals, disillusioned and at times a little frightened by the men and events over which in reality they have little control. For me, prison is a transitory affair, an experience that I could just as easily have done without; yet one in which I have discovered a number of remarkable things about my fellow man and learned much that was unknown to me before. But for Earl it is his way of life. Night- or day-shift work, five days a week, weekend overtime, condemned to watching convicts pass through the system to freedom and the hope of another life, while he remains imprisoned in a purgatory of his own choosing. For him the only escape is retirement.

"Anything exciting happen?"

"Two escapes last weekend."

"Ah!"

"Both picked up in Toronto the next day," he adds matter-of-factly in a way that indicates that their recovery is of scant personal interest.

He considers all prisoners scum. Society's dregs. None is exempt. It is only a matter of degree. I fall within the category of toleration, which is to say he will answer my questions and speak politely to me, occasionally smile. But no more.

He's a careful driver, slow and methodical. Along the way I revel silently in the sights and sounds of life. Tough-looking trucks, cold-wrapped cars with frosted windows, walkers hurrying through the chilly air. Busy movement everywhere. The tempo of life pulsating. I sit back in my seat feeling supremely happy to be alive and well and able to rejoin the game.

Kingston and environs have the highest concentration of prisons and penitentiaries of any place in North America. Divided into maximum-, medium- and minimum-security institutions, they have something for everyone. The city is an academic center too: the Royal Military College, the Canadian Armed Forces Senior Staff College, and of course Queen's University. Take away the various federal payrolls and the local economy would collapse.

In spite of the media coverage whenever a prison guard or policeman is killed in the line of duty, their jobs are among the safest in the work force. Firemen, pilots, farmers, and those working in the construction industry have a much higher percapita mortality rate. The biggest problem facing guards— "screws" to the prisoners, "correctional officers" to the general public—is boredom. The job provides little opportunity for daily exercise, requires no imagination and minimum initiative and, in time, creates a nearly comatose attitude and apathy toward the world in general.

"Have to put you in behind the walls for a couple of days," Earl states.

"Oh, why?"

"Rules."

"Ah yes. The rules."

He means that instead of taking me back to the minimum-security camp at Frontenac with its casual amenities, I will go to Collins Bay Penitentiary. Rules state that prison patients released from city hospitals must remain under observation for at least twenty-four hours in the penitentiary hospital in case medical complications develop. It is a sensible precaution, since Frontenac has neither medical staff nor facilities to cope with an emergency.

Collins Bay prison sits on a thousand acres of farmland at Kingston's western outskirts. A dreary stone-walled fortress with absurd pink-pinnacled roofs that spire over the main administration building, it looks like an abandoned movie set. A period piece from the Middle Ages. The stone, quarried from the district, is a uniformly depressing slate gray. Glass enclosed and—so I've been told by those who know—poorly heated turrets poke up from the four corners of the walls. Solitary armed guards stifled by boredom pace restlessly to keep warm, waiting for something to happen. Nothing does. After each shift they climb down the inside circular stairwell leading outside the wall and go home.

Earl delivers me through the front entrance, explaining to the uniformed guard inside the bullet-proof control center why I am here. Electrically operated steel doors motor open and we are admitted. A second guard frisks me after emptying my pockets. He isn't looking for anything: it's habit. I'm wearing civilian clothes instead of prison greens—proof that I am at the neighboring minimum-security camp and therefore not an escape risk, nor likely to be packing drugs, booze, or arms inside. And, too, I am older than the guard. There is a respect for age. Not much, but it is there. They fear the young ones, those under thirty who are still trying to prove something—macho image, strength, power, rebellion—something. Compared to them I'm a pussycat.

I stuff everything back in my pockets. The next set of steel doors whirrs open. We walk down a wide, well-lit central corridor. The hospital is the first door on the right. Earl rings for admission. Another guard appears, glances out, then unlocks. He, too, is young, regarding me warily until I smile and wish him good morning. Earl hands over my radio, personal belongings, and mumbles that he is glad I'm feeling better. He's gone before I can reply.

There are eight private rooms in the hospital, light, airy, and very clean rooms with crank-up beds, comfortable mattresses, and soft pillows. A small day room provides TV, books, radio, and kitchenette for snacks. Of course the doors are barred beyond the day room and after 10:00 P.M. the patients are locked in their rooms for the night; yet it is difficult to accept the fact that this is a prison.

A biker named Roger is hospital orderly. A tough punk with tattooed forearms that help hide the needle punctures, he's on the last few months of a ten-year sentence for armed robbery. For all his superficial toughness, wise-guy remarks and attitudes, he is strangely compassionate. His ignorance of the world is incredible. He knows little beyond this prison and is both awed and a little frightened by the imminence of his return to the world outside. He's into pills when he can get them, and speed when he can get enough to make it worthwhile to flush a vein.

He gives me his nicest room and awaits my approval and thanks before leaving. There are two others in hospital: an old man with a pacemaker that has been acting up, and a young muscular heavyweight with a damaged knee encased in a plaster cast. The old man appears spaced out and spends his time muttering oaths and obscenities to no one in particular. The heavyweight sits in his wheelchair, staring vacantly at the television and smoking endless cigarettes.

The excitement of returning to life, walking in the cold air, feeling that joy of hope for the future, has left me suddenly very tired. Before lying down I tell Roger to give my lunch to one of the others. He asks if I want my chocolate cake saved. Chocolate cake is a delicacy. Thursday lunch dessert is cake.

"Take it yourself."

In seconds I am asleep.

During the last four years I have been in and out of a variety of prisons from Los Angeles County—the worst—to the Frontenac farm camp—the best—plus a spectrum of establishments in between. It is incredible how quickly one adapts to the surroundings.

There is, of course, terror in the beginning when those steel doors clang shut with a crash of finality that sears your soul. You feel trapped. A wild animal caged. Panic fills your gorge. Vertigo. Claustrophobia. Hyperventilation. Different reactions to different personalities. I tried to ignore it all by climbing onto my narrow bunk and going to sleep. Escapism in its most basic form.

For the first weeks life becomes a succession of meals, outrage, and boredom. Long letters are written to loved ones. A sense of frustration builds at the idea of being powerless to control outside actions. The feeling of being denied the basic human needs for involvement, belonging, love, understanding, and—if you are guilty of a crime—either anger at the stupidity that led to conviction or fury at the circumstances that led to getting caught.

Gradually, as days blend into each other, your mind takes hold of the situation. Consciousness becomes concerned only with the immediate surroundings, what can be touched, seen, smelled, or tasted. Beyond this, nothing must be allowed to intrude. A period of introspection follows and you learn amazingly that freedom is a state of mind and has nothing to do with doors, bars, or prisons. Only then can the imagination be permitted once again to soar.

When I first became involved with the prison system I thought, like most people, that prisons served a useful function within society by separating the lawbreakers from the general public. I assumed that everyone in prison had been given a fair trial, found guilty, and deserved to be there. That justice was omnipotent and time spent behind bars within a prison horror was punishment at its worst and most torturous. And that upon expiration of sentence the convict would return to society's mainstream, if not reformed, certainly a good deal more cautious about his future illegal activities than when he went to jail.

Nothing could be further from the truth.

Prison is neither punitive, redemptive, nor rehabilitative. It is instead a warehousing operation designed for the benefit of those who need the system to provide their livelihood. Police, lawyers, judges, court officials, guards, parole officers, food services, social workers, and dozens of interconnecting interests that survive and thrive and grow under the criminal justice aegis.

This is not to say that I am writing a critique on how it could be run more efficiently. It is simply the way it exists today for better or worse, depending on how you view it.

But from my own observations and experiences the least benefit accrues throughout to the criminal. He is merely the faggot that fuels the financial furnace for the justice system. Perhaps this is as it should be. Yet surely there must be more practical methods for providing employment than using the human fuel of penitentiaries.

No more than 15 percent of those I met in prison needed to be there. They were the dangerous ones. The criminally insane, the double Y chromosome holders with the mad, drifting eyes who lash out with senseless murders, violent sexual assaults, or indiscriminate brutality without cause or reason. Life dealt them a busted flush at birth. Prison turns them into human debris, making them too dangerous to handle even for their guardians. If society cared they would be in mental hospitals. But society doesn't care.

Of the rest, fully 10 percent never committed the crime of which they were convicted, and shouldn't have gone to jail in the first place. The remainder could be released quite safely into society to serve their penalities in productive employment, perhaps repaying their victims and society, at least in part, for the financial costs involved in convicting them, then later doing community work best suited to their abilities. As an alternative to remaining behind bars, most would jump at the chance. On every side there are projects crying to be done for lack of people willing to work at wages that nobody will accept, while our jails are filled with idlers waiting for the years to pass.

With no shortage of leisure time I have had ample opportunity to study the system and its shortcomings. Prison libraries are crammed with books on sociology, criminology, penology, ideology, and hundreds of studies done both in and out of jails in North America about the criminal mind. Convicts write their autobiographies and are lionized by the literati and cocktail-circuit crowd, each publication offering gems of information and different viewpoints. The most interesting reading—to me at least—was in a single comparison between two annual reports provided by the Solicitor General of Canada.

For the years 1968–69 inmate population for all federal

prisons across the land amounted to 6,928 men and women. Total taxpayer's cost: 63 million dollars.

By 1979–80 that population had climbed to 9,529 souls, while the cost for keeping them behind bars jumped to a staggering 336 million dollars. Even allowing for inflation adjustment over the decade, the cost of operating the system more than quintupled. Criminal justice became a growth industry.

At last count, cost-per-inmate came to nearly $40,000 a year. From personal knowledge I know that there isn't a man within the system who wouldn't be prepared to accept half this sum in exchange for his promise to go and sin no more—and more to the point, be prepared to keep his word. Twenty thou. a year is big bread, baby. One hell of an incentive to maintain the straight and narrow.

Roger awakens me in late afternoon. No touching. That would be an invitation to retribution for assault. Instead, he shakes the bed.

"Jug-up!"

It's suppertime. Outside my window the shadows deepen. High stone walls embrace the darkness quickly. Skies blush pink, then purple, turning the stark white snow to gray.

Supper is trolleyed in from the central kitchen. Meat loaf, peas with mashed potatoes, and thick dark gravy. Tinned pears for dessert. The hospital rooms face a short day room that has been walled with thick safety glass to allow the duty guards and the nurse continuous visual contact with patients. Except for the absence of my cardiac monitor and the presence of uniformed guards, the setting is no different from the glassed fishbowl rooms in intensive care at Hotel Dieu Hospital.

We sit at a small mess table. The old man with the pacemaker shuffles out to his chair and begins shoveling in his meal; peas and gravy slobber from his spoon and chin onto the plate. Between mouthfuls he mutters fretfully, keeping his head lowered. The other two ignore him. The lad with the bum knee chews his food thoughtfully, eyes fixed on the television, lost in a world of make-believe. But then of course beyond the walls everything is make-believe. Reality is here inside prison.

Roger sits with us. He doesn't eat or watch television. Something is on his mind. One after another he drags nervously at his MacDonald's Exports, smoking them down to stubs before mashing each into a smoldering ruin. He's waiting for the others to finish and go. It's a private matter.

At last the old man belches loudly, wipes his nose on the sleeve of his nightshirt, and teeters away to the bathroom. Bumknee rolls his wheelchair in front of the television. Roger leans over the table confidentially.

"I've heard it said you write things. That true?"

He pauses a few seconds waiting for me to confirm this rumor before plunging on.

"I need a letter done to my old lady. It's worth five cartons to me—say ten if you do a real good job."

He's desperate. Inside the walls cartons of cigarettes are the exchange medium. To have a man stabbed costs only five. His hospital orderly job pays thirty dollars a month pocket money. No cash, just credit with the company store.

"I could do it myself, y'understand, but it would be much better coming from you."

"Then it wouldn't be your letter, would it?" I lower my voice level to match his so that the others can't pick up on our conversation.

"Sure it would. I'll tell you what to say. You clean up the words, spelling—that sort of thing. You can do that, can't you? I mean, I got no education. Grade six that's all. I can read and write, but not that good. Bev—the old lady—she's got grade twelve. I don't want her to remember me as a dummy."

Every wife, girl friend, or mistress is called "my old lady." There is a special need to possess a woman, if only in imagination.

"Once I came inside, we sorta fell out of touch. My kid will be nine this summer. I've never seen him. She sent me a picture a few years back. What could I say? Nothing. I never answered."

Does every father dream of his son? The son who will

become all the things he could never be, with all the attributes he could never acquire, reaching those pinnacles he could never attain? It must be a basic paternal ingredient in all of us. I understand.

Roger explains that they lived with her folks on a farm outside Brantford. Mickey, his son, should be in grade four now if he managed to pass his first three years.

"Do they flunk kids that young if they fuck up?" he asks earnestly, expecting the worst.

As I finish my pears he tells of the happy times with his old lady. Summer evenings in a distant August with the air warm and mellow, the sounds of frogs and crickets floating in chorus from her father's irrigation pond. Laughter and love under a billion stars in a ripening field. Such memories have sustained him through long lonely years. Memories and a tattered snapshot of a naked infant.

It would be too crass for me to inquire the basis for his assuming that both wife and child are still interested in hearing from him, much less seeing him again. Maybe Bev has remarried, delivered more children, left the farm when her parents died to live in California with a big burly husband who chews up tattooed motorcycle punks and swallows the pieces. But for Roger the intervening wasted years don't count. Time stopped the day he went inside.

I promise to write his letter. I don't need his cigarette cartons, but rather than place him in a position where he owes me a favor, I'll take them. That way we stay even. In prison it's important to stay even with everyone. Nobody likes favors owing or owed.

Before he can start the letter the duty guard sticks his head in the door and calls. I have a visitor.

Unlike the easy atmosphere at a minimum-security institution, the Collins Bay visiting area has tightly controlled and monitored access. Its visiting room is cramped and crowded, the walls lined with coin-operated food and drink machines and an assortment of scruffy chairs containing even scruffier-looking people. The air is close and a little smelly. Helen looks lost amid this human debris. It is the first time she has been inside a real prison like this one. Her face mirrors her surprise at the discovery of conditions. We sit holding hands like juveniles.

"I didn't bring the children," she apologizes.

"Just as well. No point in exposing them to this along with everything else."

They have come to see me only in Frontenac, where the visiting room with its casual openness and general congeniality is quite different from the noisy, abrasive atmosphere inside Collins Bay. Here, visitors and prisoners are literally shoe-horned into the cramped quarters. Privacy or soft, confiding conversation is impossible. It is intended to be. At Frontenac, during the summer, outdoor visits are encouraged. Picnic tables and a children's playground provide a feeling of family intimacy without the constricting and all-pervading presence of uni-formed guards. Here, observers ensconced behind thick bullet-proof glass see everything.

Well, not quite everything. Seated nearby, a young woman with her back to the guards gives her man a hand job during a long, loving embrace. He flinches on the glory stroke. Her handkerchief covers his sticky emission. She wipes him gently, then stuffs the handkerchief into her blouse. No one pays them the least attention, whether from courtesy or indifference is difficult to say. Helen watches, fascinated. Children scamper past.

"You're staring. It isn't nice to stare."

"God what a place! It's a Carnival of Animals."

Not really. For anyone not used to seeing frustrated human emotions satisfied in public by necessity, the revelation comes as a shock. We consider sex and love and public displays of affection to be coarse, things that should be conducted in private. But when the law in its wisdom condemns one of the partners to prison, what is the alternative? Human beings require emo-tional release to bind them. For every man punished through imprisonment there is usually an innocent woman, and often several innocent children, who are being punished as well. It is the way we have designed our system.

In such an atmosphere Helen finds it difficult to speak of anything. I am sorry she came, sorry to have subjected her to this spectacle. She looks frightened. I squeeze her hand.

"Cheer up, sweetheart. In fifty years none of this will even survive as memory."

Today this is a small consolation for either one of us.

Visiting hours are from six until eight. After fifteen minutes I shoo her out. She doesn't protest. A final wave and she's gone. After another perfunctory search, another sliding steel door, I am returned to the hospital.

Roger has finished the first page of what he wants to send to his old lady. It's penciled on a lined copybook page. His scrawl is big and childish and filled with spelling mistakes—phonetic English as its worst. He watches my expression closely while I read his effort. It is pathetic.

Hey there babie.
Bet you never thout youd here from yore old man agin did you now? Well here I am big as life and twice as ungly. How is the kid? How are you? I am OK. Getting outa here soon. Like to see you and our kid. Gess you have changed. I have changed to. Everibody changes. Know what I mean? Mabe we kan get it on agin like it usta be. Remember? Stay cool. Roger.

His eyes hold a tortured look because he knows that the letter is terrible but he can't find the words to explain his feelings. So long has he suppressed them in order to maintain his phony macho bike-hog image, he's forgotten how to express sorrow, regret, apology, and love.

"It's not very good, I know. But that's the sort of thing I want to say. You put it into nicer words for me. I'll check back in the morning. Maybe you'll get a couple of ideas, eh?"

Embarrassed, he collects the supper dishes and rolls the serving table back to the kitchens. After he's gone I tear his letter into tiny pieces and take a fresh page from the scribbler.

My Dearest Beverly,
Time passes. I grow older and wiser. The years blend into

each other. Soon I shall be leaving this place forever, God willing. If you can forgive the hurt, the pain, the sadness I have left with you I would like to do something for you and our son— if you'll let me.

This poem says it much better than I can.

I will make you brooches and toys for your delight
Of bird-song at morning and star-shine at night.
I will make a palace fit for you and me,
Of green days in forests and blue days at sea.

I will make my kitchen, and you shall keep your
*   room,*
Where white flows the river and bright blows the
*   bloom,*
And you shall wash your linen and keep your body
*   white*
In rainfall at morning and dewfall at night.

And this shall be for music when no one else is
*   near,*
The fine song for singing, the rare song to hear!
That only I remember, that only you admire,
Of the broad road that stretches and the roadside
*   fire.*

Please write when you have time.

It is very short, but more than enough for what he needs. Besides, I am tired again. After a leisurely shower, I brush my teeth and climb into bed. I hear neither the guard locking my door nor the half-hour rounds throughout the long winter night. The room is cooled and heated through an overhead duct. Something is wrong with the system: by morning my teeth are chattering. The room's temperature has plunged to near freezing and cold air continues to flow from the ceiling. The duty guards apologize when they unlock our doors.

Roger rolls in the breakfast trolley. Inside the cabinet he has stacked five cartons of cigarettes. He delivers them to my room and takes the letter. He reads it once, twice. His eyes fill and he blinks to clear the moisture. It is not what he had expected. He mutters a gruff thanks and promises to send me another five cartons in the laundry pickup.

Doctor Ted DeJager turns up midmorning oozing with sympathetic concern and an uncustomary degree of willingness to offer me any amount of personal and professional assistance, from letters to the Parole Board and Frontenac staff relieving me from prison duties to visiting Helen with the very latest update on my physical condition. I have to give him credit. He's trying to make amends. And he has a lot of amends to make.

He draws me confidentially away from the others to explain that there are so many fuck-offs inside that it's hard to know when he's getting a straight story or a line of bullshit. He figures that if he took everyone's word on face value, most of the prison population would be lying on their collective asses in hospital. As it is, half of the bastards probably slip past him with imaginary illnesses.

What is the point of arguing with him? Yet isn't a doctor supposed to know if a patient is sick or bluffing through those vital signs of heart, chest sounds, lungs, eyes, pressure, throat, skin and fingernail coloration? Or are those ritualistic and methodical examinations merely a form of juju?

The nurse gives me several packages of pills from the pharmacy, including a small brown bottle of nitroglycerin tablets in case of recurring angina pains. They are Dr. Koval's prescriptions: Inderal, Anturan, and Digoxin. Dosages and the times they are to be taken have been written on each brown packet. At this rate I will become a pillhead.

Bill Briscoe appears with his Frontenac deliveries. One man hobbling on crutches, his foot encased in bandages, is here for a change of dressings. Another is in for the removal of seven stitches in his scalp following a farm accident the previous week. These prisoners are dressed in civilian clothes, blue jeans, sports shirts, and wool sweaters. Only their footwear and parkas are government issue. Convicts prefer to stay out of prison greens whenever they can manage it. In the hospital waiting room the

Frontenac visitors are regarded enviously by the Collins Bay crowd of malingerers, all waiting to see Ted DeJager with their stories. I join them and sit and wait.

"You going to live, Foster?" Briscoe demands.

"Forever."

I like Briscoe. In fact I like him better than any prison guard, counselor, classification officer, or parole officer I've encountered. He is a tall, slim man with an agreeable stoop and wide, humorous eyes that regard the world as pure sitcom, written and performed for his enjoyment. He treats everybody with the same courtesy, inmates and staff alike. No favorites, never a condemnation, a sympathetic man with a golden heart. If only they were all like Briscoe.

His hobby is old cars: restoring the past to perfection with skillful hands. Occasionally he arrives at work in one of these gems to set tongues wagging in admiration and derision.

While we wait Briscoe tells me about his heart attack. He was at the minimum-security camp near Petawawa three years before. They rushed him by ambulance into Ottawa. He still carries nitro pills.

"See?"

It is a duplicate of my own bottle.

"Did the angina pains come back?"

"A few months later—not as bad, but bad enough," he allows.

"Mine are gone."

"They'll be back," he says sadly. "Main thing is never to let yourself get too excited about anything. That's when it really hits me. Just relax and let the world slide by."

When the nurse and doctor have finished their work Briscoe takes all of us out the back exit to his van.

We drive within the walls to the rear gate, stopping on the way to pick up our laundry sacks. Regulations require the van to stop three hundred feet from the gate and the driver to climb out, showing the guards in the towers and reception office that he is not being held hostage. Briscoe holds up his arms, then slides back in the seat. At the gate we stop once more. Everyone climbs out while van and passengers are searched again for contraband. It's a foolish exercise looking under the hood, peering at the motor, under the frame, inside the wheel wells. No one ever thinks to check the laundry bags going in or out of Collins Bay. Why spoil a good mailing system?

After shakedown we're allowed to proceed beyond the steel gates for the quarter-mile drive along the prison's rear wall to the freedom of Frontenac and noonday lunch with five choices of dessert. This is jail?

Woodstock, Canada

25 March 1979

By noon on Sunday both police and prosecutor are beginning to look worried that things might not turn out exactly as planned. Mac Haig, our reporter from the *London Free Press*, says that there's an old adage in jurisprudence which claims that the longer juries remain closeted, the less likely they will reach a verdict favorable to the prosecution, or indeed any verdict at all. Ours has been out for three days. But I am not optimistic.

Defense and prosecution alike sit smoking or pacing the wide, creaking corridors in the old Oxford County courthouse. Outside in the sunny spring day the snow has nearly gone and on the broad, sloping lawns tiny leafy shoots poke up with seasonal energy. But indoors, time has taken a deep breath and stopped to await a verdict from ten men and one woman. One juror, a farmer, was excused to plant his crop before the trial ended. Like a heavy lead plumb, suspense hangs over the cigarette smoke and desultory conversation. With the contest ended, the protagonists need no longer posture. Even the judge comes from his chambers on Mount Olympus to sit in the corridor with the rabble and puff his pipe reflectively. Jim Riley, the chief investigating officer, tries to ingratiate himself with his honor in stilted discussion. Together they make an interesting pair: the Pride and Prejudice of Justice.

Judge Chester Misner is a wiry, combative little man with angular features and a sharp nose. His temper is quick, his mind agile. I have become convinced that he has been given orders to get a conviction in whatever way he can. (Irrationally, I am suspicious of everything and everyone. Criminal trials have a way of doing this to defendants. It's no fun being in the hot seat.) Since the trial began in January he has interrupted proceedings 528 times by actual count, either to berate the defense, to challenge witnesses' testimony whenever it appeared to be benefiting the accused, or to provide gratuitous commentary throughout the trial, leaving little doubt in the defendants' minds as to the verdict he expected the jury to return.

Until now I did not realize the ease with which a judge can influence the course of a trial, should he decide to exchange his role of impartial referee for assistant prosecutor. Although Misner's been three years on the bench, this is his first criminal trial in which two of the three defendants are forced to act without benefit of counsel. This, too, I suspect, has been planned by higher authority to insure conviction.

Emotionally and physically I am drained. For too long I have been gobbling tablets for indigestion, Valiums to steady my nerves, sitting up late every night smoking endless cigarettes and planning the next day's courtroom tactics. All have taken their toll. I'm wrecked. I'd like to run away to a white sandy beach I remember in the Yucatan. I would lie in mindless torpor under emerald skies, watching gulls reel, children playing on the warm sand. Peace.

"It looks like you're going to walk, Tony," Riley says as I pass the yellow oak bench where he and Misner are seated.

"Are you serious?"

But I can see from his eyes that he means it. Impossible. Has he missed what the judge did to the jury, or have I become totally paranoid? Riley looks uneasy, perhaps a bit fearful that his five-year pursuit and million-dollar case has come to nothing. A verdict of "not guilty." Wouldn't it be nice?

Misner puffs his pipe, his eyes opaque, his smile knowing. We understand each other perfectly. My whole problem has been that Riley is a naïve, stubborn bulldog. Is it so difficult for him to see that, regardless of what verdict the jury return, he has won already? The day that he and his army of policemen seized my company records five years ago was when I lost the game.

It began innocuously enough to satisfy any writer of melodrama. Two neighbours talking over the back fence, discussing an investment that one of them had made the previous winter in an improbable-sounding Brazilian gold bullion scheme. The second neighbor was a policeman. He reported his conversation to the local Oxford County Crown Attorney, Fred Porter, who in turn passed the matter on to Ontario Provincial Police Headquarters in Toronto. Corporal Jim Riley, promoted up from highway patrol to Anti-rackets, was given the investigation. It was his second day on the job.

For six months Riley and his men played a game of cops and robbers in the best textbook tradition. All Midair company principals—past and present—were placed under surveillence. Investor meetings were scoped through telephoto lenses; wire taps were installed on a variety of phones. Wherever I drove or flew I had an escort, either a few car lengths behind on the highway or a few seats back on the airline. Had it not been for the ultimate devastating effect of their efforts, it might have been uproariously funny, for there were certainly elements of comic opera to the whole business. I know of no group of people in society who take themselves more seriously than policemen, irrespective of the absurdities they are ordered to undertake in the name of the law.

While I raced to complete the financing with undercover policemen in close pursuit I hoped that they had sense enough to realize through their eavesdropping that I was doing nothing illegal. But it was not to be and to this day I am convinced that it was the threat of my success that persuaded Riley to act and seize the company's records while I was in California. He had spent too much time and money on men and equipment by then to let it slip away. Investors who make substantial profits tend to make poor prosecution witnesses in fraud trials, regardless of any charges made by the police.

I flew back from California as soon as my brother called me, and made arrangements to meet Riley. For a week he stonewalled. Too busy. Out of town on other business. Finally, after several phone calls from my lawyer, a meeting was set at one of their local traffic divisions in Toronto. Riley arrived with an experienced police interrogator, Sergeant Carl Manneke. I brought my lawyer. We talked.

The meeting was useful to the extent that I learned there

was little likelihood of getting the company's books and records returned in the foreseeable future, and that the police believed they had uncovered the largest international crime organization in Canada since the rum-running Thirties. In their eyes every activity in which Midair and its directors had been engaged smacked of fraud. Not little-old-lady swindles, but the type that cause governments to collapse, wars to commence, and public chaos. It was too bizarre to be believed. Yet they believed it. In their eyes that made it fact. Police logic.

"When do I get the company's books returned?"

"A few weeks. Give us a chance to go over them, Tony."

Manneke was very chummy. First names for everyone. No point standing on formalities. Riley sat looking glum.

"Are you going to do an audit?"

"A complete audit will be done," he promised.

That was good news if it was true. A complete audit would cost me at least ten thousand dollars, and had to be done before concluding either the German financing or the British management agreement. Far better that the police pay for it than I.

Later, in a coffee shop on the way back into town, my lawyer laughed: "An audit? Those two couldn't read a balance sheet if their lives depended on it. It'll never happen."

Harry Kerr is a lawyer with a business mind. Four weeks earlier I had taken him to England for the final touches to my negotiations with Keegan. Harry had made the deal with Keegan work. Now Riley had seized his records too.

"You want it straight?" he asked, stirring his coffee.

"Of course."

"Get yourself a criminal lawyer. A good one. The police have ninety days to shit or get off the pot. After that they'll either give the books back—unaudited—or arrest you for fraud. I'm betting on your arrest. You have about three months to cover your ass."

"But, Harry, there is no fraud! No one has scammed anything. There are no secret Swiss accounts. I didn't join the jet set. They've got to find out eventually that it's legitimate! Maybe Riley figures I'm his ticket to stardom, but no one has done anything wrong. You know that."

"What's that got to do with it? If they think you're guilty of something, you are guilty. If they want your ass nailed to the crossbars, that's what's going to happen to you and anyone else they decide should swing with you. It may be tough, but that's justice. I didn't invent the system."

Almost three months to the day after the search warrants were executed, Riley arrested Eric Schwendau, Angelo Guglielmo, an Italian contractor, and me for fraud. It made front-page headlines in the regional papers and inside pages of the national dailies. The stories had enough to titillate the most jaded news junkie: illegal diamonds, surplus warplanes for Pakistan, stolen stock certificates and securities with Mafia overtones, hundreds of millions' worth of gold bullion to be lifted from Brazil to Zurich, and the novelty of four-motored crop dusters flying about the world.

The Crown Prosecutor, Fred Porter, took the position that every financial transaction had been a carefully planned fraud designed by the accused to enrich themselves. But, from the standpoint of global politics and business intrigues, Porter knew little about the real world beyond Oxford County. He was taking every bit from Riley as gospel.

Guglielmo and I were transported from London to the holding cells outside Woodstock. Schwendau arrived a little later with an escort from Toronto. We spent a good part of the evening analyzing the absurdity of the situation, calling to one another from our respective cells. No provision had been made for feeding us, so we paid for our own supper, which was brought in by a sympathetic cop from one of the local fast-food outlets.

In the morning, accompanied by news reporters and photographers, we appeared before the local Woodstock magistrate to be charged formally. The bail was based on our collective undertakings to appear for all subsequent court appearances, turn in our passports, and—oddly—refrain from contacting any of the Crown's witnesses or our company investors until the trial date. We signed the necessary promissory papers and drove home.

Helen and the children were in a frightful state of emotional turmoil. The Foster family had become social lepers overnight. For youngsters in grade school, being told that their father was a crook and a murderer who was going to be sent to the electric chair comes as a tremendous shock. Children can be very cruel to their peers who suffer physical handicaps or public outrage. Even Helen had received a variety of taunting phone calls the night after the evening newscasts. My first instinct was to shield them from the limelight. I considered alternatives. We could sell the house and move to another part of the country where Ontario Provincial Police dementia would be regarded with scant interest. I could return for the periodic appearances at court and stay with Guglielmo during the trial, still months away. At least Helen and the children would then be spared. This was not their fight. Why should they be made to suffer? I was still naïve enough to believe that I could win in a court of law.

In the end I did nothing, for within a week the publicity had died and for the time being I had become yesterday's news. Best of all, the children's playmates decided that their father wasn't going to get the chair after all. Things gradually returned to normal, at least on the surface. Underneath, menace hung over every waking hour like a Damoclean sword.

Of course my German investors and British management agreements dissolved in a North Sea mist once I advised of the company's inability to produce an audited financial report, owing to the police seizures.

For the first weeks after the seizures I hustled across the country for another investor. In Calgary I ran into Sydney Williams, an ex-CPR railroad detective from Montreal who had struck it rich with a car leasing business in Los Angeles. He was prepared to pick up in part where the Germans and Brits had left off, consolidating Midair's assets under one roof and corporate structure.

Interact Aircraft of America opened its office at Burbank Airport in the San Fernando Valley during early July. Everything left from the Midair mess at the Daggett Airport in the

Mojave was moved by truck and air to beautiful downtown Burbank.

Once Riley caught wind of what was happening, he informed Williams that the entire Midair concept was a massive fraud and that I would probably be arrested shortly. If Sydney didn't want to put himself under suspicion as well, he would be best advised to steer clear. But Williams didn't scare that easily. At least not then.

One of the bail conditions specified that if I wanted to go to the States on business, I must notify Riley of my departure time, destination, and itinerary. It seemed a pointless exercise and one designed more for harassment than for fulfillment of any legal function. But on my first trip away from home I discovered another reason for this addendum to my bail conditions.

Landing in California two weeks later, I was met at the airport by officers of the Border Patrol, Sheriff's Department, and the FBI, all armed to the teeth and regarding me very warily. I was given a professional frisking, uncomfortably handcuffed, and slung into the back seat of a cop car. We drove at breakneck speed to the local county jail. The warrants issued consisted of my being an "undesirable alien." Oddly, these American cops had a full report on the Woodstock affair, even to a copy of the charges.

For two days I waited, subsisting on frightful bologna sandwiches washed down by a sweet, muddy liquid that the jail advertised as "cowfee." Williams bailed me out on the third day by posting $3,000 cash. Just in the nick of time, too, for I was due in Woodstock the next afternoon for what turned out to be a nearly endless session of monthly postponements of my court case while a preliminary hearing date was decided.

Although Riley professed total ignorance of my U.S. arrest, I learned later from the California Border Patrol that the orders had originated from their Buffalo immigration office after a request had been received from the "Canadian police in Toronto."

During August I flew with Williams between New York, the World Bank in Washington, and Burbank trying to make the new company as painless a transition from Midair to Interact as possible. Williams agreed to honor all Midair debts out of eventual profits through the device of using me as sole creditor for the new company. Now contracts appeared from World Bank and there was a rush to get the aircraft into immediate operation.

A new and more efficient navigational system for the DC-7 had appeared during the summer. Produced by Global Navigation, Inc., of Torrance, California, the new units were half the price and twice the accuracy of the INS system used in Quebec three years earlier. Several state and federal forestry officials wanted to see the newer system operate under simulated spraying conditions. However, instead of using the costly DC-7 for these demonstrations, Williams wanted me to find a smaller, less expensive machine to operate. As president and chief executive officer of Interact he intended to keep a tight rein on expenses.

While I was looking, Williams's Beverly Hills attorney suggested a short-term lease with one of his clients, Charlie Hudson, who operated several twin-engined Beechcraft ten-place aircraft. Sixty dollars an hour instead of six hundred. The economics were right. The aircraft, unfortunately, wasn't. His client was operating a Mexican marijuana-smuggling operation.

On the morning of September 4 while waiting for our leased Beechcraft to arrive from Culiacan, I managed to get myself arrested for a third time in as many weeks. No mean feat.

Shortly after the machine landed at a deserted ranch airstrip in the mountains east of Ventura, a posse of narcs from the Drug Enforcement Administration charged down from the hills in three high-speed cars and, after waving a variety of weapons and warrants in everybody's face, arrested the lot of us as we stood waiting in the cool morning air. But they missed one man.

The aircraft's pilot had gone over to one of the abandoned sheds nearby to defecate after his nonstop nine-hour trip. When he saw the cars coming he pulled his pants up quickly and clambered onto the building's rafters, where he remained for the next seven hours under its broiling tin roof until police vacated the area.

The rest of us were handcuffed, lined up on our knees, then one by one taken apart from the others to be interrogated. Both sides looked very young, clean cut, and not at all what one might visualize as heavy-duty criminals or law enforcement officers. Yet the narcs appeared far more nervous and ill at ease than the smugglers, and kept looking anxiously toward the surrounding hills as if expecting reinforcements to arrive and tip the balance against them.

As the oldest of the group and wearing aviation sunglasses I was a natural for the choice of pilot. When I admitted that I was indeed licensed to fly, that cinched it. I tried to explain the purpose of my presence, the aircraft-leasing arrangements, the ferry trip to Burbank for navigational testing. All of it could easily be verified by a phone call to Sydney Williams. But it was no use. *Numero Uno* for this smuggling operation had been found to their satisfaction: me. I was sent back to join the others.

A helicopter fluttered down nearby. Mr. Big emerged, ducking his head beneath the rotor blades. He strutted up and down the line of kneeling men, making silly threats and shouting hoarsely. Overhead, a DEA Mohawk surveillence aircraft swooped low and waggled its wings as if its crew had been responsible for the entire scene on the ground below.

After several hours of waiting uncomfortably in a progressively hotter day, we were loaded aboard two paddy wagons that arrived from San Luis Obispo to take us to the county jail. More bologna sandwiches and lukewarm "cowfee."

The charges were the same for everyone: "conspiracy to transport a controlled substance into the U.S." My bail was set at ten thousand dollars. Williams's attorney arranged the payment through a local bondsman and I was on my way back to Canada the following afternoon for the next Woodstock appearance.

Riley, meanwhile, had been promoted to sergeant and given an increased expense allocation to find some hard evidence for the upcoming preliminary hearing. He decided to visit the States with an accountant to check out the authenticity of Midair's former operations at Daggett Airport. After a long, imaginative tale to one local San Bernardino County judge, he obtained a search warrant and drove out to the airport with two sheriff's men. Midair's U.S. books and records were locked in a trailer. No problem. They smashed the door, locks, filing cabinets, and loaded anything that looked interesting into their car.

Later, upon examination, there turned out to be little of value—certainly nothing convincing enough to prove that Midair Inc. had been anything other than a legitimate business. However, while in California he did hear about my San Luis Obispo arrest and the smuggling charges.

He returned to Canada at once and arranged a "show cause hearing" to have my bail canceled and so keep me on ice in jail until trial. At the speed with which Canadian justice moved, this would have meant years of sitting in enforced idleness. The hearing was set for late November.

A frantic travel and work regimen began, far more intense than anything I'd experienced with Midair. Between costly and totally wasteful courtroom appearances in Woodstock and Los Angeles for my two pending trials, I continued to work at top speed to turn Interact into a functioning corporation. Maintenance and flight crews were hired and trained at the Burbank facility. Testing was done in the mountains and desert nearby. There were a number of bids to prepare for spray work in the states of Maine, Florida, Louisiana, Washington, and California, plus continuation of the global negotiations that Midair had originally initiated elsewhere in the world. Finally there were the two defense positions to prepare for the lawyers hired to represent me. Rarely was I at home for more than a few hours as I raced to complete these business arrangements in case the worst should happen.

The show cause hearing was held in November, but the judge ruled that, since I had not yet been convicted of anything, there had to be a presumption of innocence. Sydney Williams's presence and testimony cinched it. My bail was continued as before.

By December Williams had either arranged for or purchased the last of Midair's assets from creditors. On New Year's Day, 1976, I took off from London Airport with the last DC-7 that had been grounded by creditor's litigation. It was an embarrassment to the police, who had maintained that the aircraft was so badly mauled and decayed that it would never fly again. I landed it at Burbank Airport two days later and went to see a doctor.

Chest pains had been plaguing me over the preceding months. I was experiencing shortness of breath coupled with what felt like acute indigestion whenever I drove myself too hard. Heart problems were the last thing to cross my mind. The doctor, an FAA medical inspector, gave me a pilot's license-renewal examination and identified the chest pain as nervous indigestion brought about by the number of cigarettes I was smoking.

"Cut down your smoking and you'll feel much better. Or switch to a pipe."

Sure. First thing tomorrow morning.

The next hurdle came during late February. While I had been absorbed with the business of Interact, a series of wheeling and dealing had been going on behind the scenes with the Los Angeles D.A.'s office. A few days before the trial I learned that the main prosecution witnesses were to be the owner of the smuggling operation and his partner. In exchange for probationary sentences they had agreed to testify against everyone else, myself included.

Horrified, I drove out to Ventura and called on Charles Hudson. He operated "Charmin' Charlie's" golf driving range at the city's outskirts and held a PGA instructor's license, boasting among his friends such notables as James Garner and Efrem Zimbalist, Jr., both of whom he had taught to improve their swing.

After hearing my supplication Hudson merely shrugged his fat shoulders and apologized by saying that he couldn't be expected to turn in the man who had actually flown his aircraft and managed to escape because the fellow was already free on bail for a similar charge and, additionally, on parole for the same offense. A man in his mid-sixties, if he were to be nailed again on another smuggling charge the court would put him away forever.

"Tough," I roared. "But where does that leave me, you rotten sonofabitch?"

"Oh, you'll figure something out when the time comes. Why not jump bail? Who is going to chase you back to Canada?"

I swore to fight him in court.

"Then you'll lose," he told me without rancor.

My lawyer, Steve Heiser, charged ten thousand dollars for what turned out to be a one-day trial. The other defendants, with one exception, used novice attorneys from the Public Defender's Office, a vast legal pool providing a living wage for apprentice lawyers while they practiced with courtroom cadavers.

Hudson and his partner sat in the back of the courtroom with smarmy smiles for anyone willing to look in their direction. The young assistant D.A. in charge of the case held a conference with the rest of the lawyers to offer a deal once the DEA agents had testified. Things weren't quite as open and shut as they appeared.

If the defendants would plead guilty, hizzonor would award minimal sentences to everyone. In California, marijuana wasn't considered much of a crime in 1976. Judge Irving Hill, we learned, was anxious to get on with a more important case, involving movie actor Robert Cummings and Pacific Telephone, which was next on his court docket. Marijuana trials bored him, his clerk explained; hence this offer to the defendants. So, was everybody prepared to accept this gesture of judicial munificence in the interests of speedy justice?

They certainly were. All except one. I refused flatly on the basis of my innocence and because a criminal record would bar me from re-entering the United States. Heiser agreed and returned to huddle with the assistant D.A. while I sat under a storm of stony stares from the other defendants. Three-month sentences for a ton of Mexican weed sounded fine to them. For me it would be disaster. I was due in Woodstock on Monday to start the preliminary hearing. I intended to be there.

After much discussion a compromise was found between the court and the lawyers. If the accused would sign a "statement of fact" recognizing the prosecution's position, but without pleading guilty to the charges, the judge would agree to release everyone after conviction and let the appeal court decide on the validity of the arrests and charges. The DEA, it seemed, had violated a number of civil rights in the method by which their case had been conducted. Heiser was satisfied that an appeal would reverse all convictions, in effect canceling out the entire affair.

"What's the alternative?" I inquired.

He shook his head. "Jury trial. Twelve men and women tried and true who will convict you after the judge finishes lecturing them on the immorality of demon weed. For a first offense you'll get the maximum: five years. I recommend that you take his deal."

Thus I arrived back in Woodstock on an appeal bond with a smuggling conviction hanging over my head. Riley met me in the courtroom corridor and gave a huge crocodile smile.

"Are you interested in talking a deal for my case now?"

"No."

"I can afford to wait. The time will come."

Maddeningly, he oozed confidence, although two weeks later when the hearing was over, his confidence had evaporated.

Preliminary hearings are designed to provide the defense with an opportunity to learn what sort of case the prosecution has going for it. A courtroom "show and tell." If the prosecution's case is obviously too weak to take to trial, the presiding judge may decide to dismiss the proceedings, although the prosecutor is never duty-bound to accept this decision.

After listening to the Crown attorney present his evidence for a week and a half, and with another week left to go, my lawyer, Robert Carter, suggested that we end the agony. In his opinion the Crown had no case but the Crown attorney had made it clear that, regardless of the judge's recommendations, he intended to go to trial. Why waste further legal fees?

All defendants elected to go to trial at once. Startled, Fred

Porter began fudging for delay, suggesting a September date as being most convenient for the Crown. This convenience would provide Riley with more time to get out and dig up some hard evidence. So far, everything offered had been circumstantial.

During the rest of the spring and summer months I kept a very low business profile. Williams wanted me to stay well away from company activities until both the U.S. appeal and the Woodstock trial had been satisfactorily concluded. For some time he'd been under increasing pressure and intimidation from police in both countries to drop the Interact, Inc., operations completely and anything else connected with me. I was considered now to be a kingpin in the global drug-trafficking scene.

It was decided that I should devote my time to preparing for the upcoming trial, now only five months away. After weeks of research and written preparation, the time came for travel abroad for foreign witnesses. Visits to Venezuela and Brazil were necessary after several long-distance phone calls had failed to convince our former associates that their presence was mandatory for our acquittal. On Riley's instructions I sent a traveling request to his boss, Superintendent Peter Sawaski, asking for my passport and explaining the purpose of my trips.

While I was awaiting a reply, Heiser phoned from California with the startling news that Judge Hill wanted me back in his court the following Monday for a show cause hearing to revoke my appeal bond. He had received word that I was planning an escape to Brazil!

Checkmate.

I explained what was going to happen as best I could to Helen, kissed the children good-by, and caught a flight to Los Angeles, hoping that U.S. immigration would refuse me entry. No such luck.

Although Riley was in L.A., he didn't appear in court. Instead, his statement was read into the record by the prosecutor, along with my letter to Sawaski, both given as *prima-facie* proof of my intent to skip out from Judge Hill's marijuana conviction. Anything I had to say fell on deaf ears.

Heiser shook his head and apologized for not having recognized this danger from Canadian police influences sooner, after I had warned him what might happen.

Bail was revoked and I was ordered to begin serving a fifteen-month sentence at the federal prison on Terminal Island. The irony of it was laughable. While the others who had been convicted remained free on appeal bonds and continued working at their questionable profession, I went to jail for trying to gather witnesses and prove innocence in another case. Wheels within wheels within wheels. The joke was on me.

Terminal Island had been the U.S. Navy's prison stockade during World War II. The island, sandwiched in between the cities of San Pedro and Long Beach, provided dock facilities for the Coast Guard, a fleet of tuna boats, and Howard Hughes's huge *Glomar Explorer*.

The prison, situated next to the Coast Guard Station at the island's western tip, had been designated for an experiment in mixed sex cohabitation. A hundred female prisoners wearing normal street clothes mingled freely with six hundred khaki-clad male convicts during waking hours at work, meals, and leisure time. Sandra Good, one of the Manson flower children, was there, along with Sarah Jane Moore, who had tried to assassinate President Gerald Ford the previous year. Before my release I got to know them quite well, although never well enough to understand their peculiar philosophies. Perhaps I was too thick-headed to appreciate the subtle nuances of anarchy.

Oddly, I enjoyed my eight-month stay at T.I. The weather was beautiful, the food superb, amusements and movies free, the surrounding company fascinating, and for the first time in many years I was under no financial or business pressures. To pass the time I began writing a novel, finishing it the week before my release.

Although I was under no pressure, Helen was going through a financial hell and one of the worst winters on record in Canada. To pay the bills she took in a university student boarder and found herself a job selling kinky lingerie at a local porno shop. It didn't pay much but she got to meet a lot of weird people. The children learned to make their own lunches at noon and get back to school on time. They responded magnificiently to the situation.

The prison provided twenty-four-hour-a-day telephone access for inmate use. Keeping in touch through that "long-distance feeling" was never a problem, but from a practical standpoint there was little I could do to help the family situation, and lengthy collect calls only served to add additional crushing expense. We kept them to one ten-minute call a week. Little enough, but it had to do.

In April I was released from prison to serve the rest of my sentence in virtual freedom at a halfway house in Long Beach. Interact had disappeared with my incarceration. Williams lost interest when the employees looted the equipment and aircraft. He moved to Calgary and never returned. Helen flew down to visit and we spent a happy weekend catching up. But by July Riley learned that I was free and the L.A. authorities received word from their Canadian brethren that I was planning an escape from the halfway house. Accordingly, the last three weeks of my sentence were spent in maximum security back at Terminal Island. This time I did laugh because I no longer cared.

From Terminal Island immigration officers picked me up and dropped me at the L.A. County jail, where I waited another three weeks for extradition proceedings and an escort from the Ontario police to arrive and take me home. The former I waived as being absurd; the latter I rather enjoyed because the plainclothes officer kept me entertained all the way home on Air Canada. Once back, I was deposited into the local Middlesex County Detention Center to await another bail hearing. By this time Helen and the children were visiting her parents on the East Coast and managed to miss this part of the insanity.

The hearing resulted in my being released. I seemed to have much better luck with Canadian bail hearings than with those in the States. Maybe Ontario judges were less impressed by police testimony than their American counterparts.

Our house had been put up for sale, most of its furnishings already sold at public auction. I borrowed a car and went looking for rental accommodation close to Woodstock so that Helen and the children would have a place to return to at the start of the school year. In the quiet town of Ingersoll I found a modest townhouse, but the police refused to allow me to fly into Halifax and drive my family home. I accepted Guglielmo's offer to go in my place.

Angelo Guglielmo had arrived in Canada in the early 1950s when English classes for immigrants were nonexistent. Over the years he forgot most of his Italian and never learned proper English. Although nearly inarticulate in both languages, he had a heart of gold. His only crime, so far as I could determine, had been in trying to help Schwendau and me to finance Midair by investing money in the company. He understood very little about the more than thirty charges against him but, like me, was completely convinced of his innocence and what the outcome of any jury trial would be.

The trial opened in early November. G. Stewart McKeown, a charming Toronto attorney, represented Schwendau through Legal Aid. Harold Stafford Q.C. spoke for Guglielmo while I, reluctantly, acted for myself. My attempts to obtain Legal Aid services had been refused on the grounds that I should use some of the vast sums of money I had squirreled away in offshore banks! Oh, that this had been true.

For weeks, then months, the trial lumbered forward to the delight and amusement of southwestern Ontario newspaper readers. In addition to an assortment of Canadians, witnesses came from everywhere: Brazil, Venezuela, the United States, Italy, England. Heady times for the Grand Duchy of Oxford County. The cost must have been enormous.

There was a brief Christmas recess, then everybody was back in court for more weeks of comedy and intrigue. Finally, near the middle of February, the Crown rested its case. And not a moment too soon. To the defense it was obvious what the verdict would be even before presenting our side of the case. Of course the Crown attorney realized this too. What to do? A "not guilty" verdict would make the attorney general's department a laughing-stock, and subject to all sorts of nasty civil litigation. An adjournment was called by the Crown to sort things out.

When court reconvened on the last day of February it was to announce a mistrial. Harold Stafford, who had been dismissed as counsel by Guglielmo on February 16 after having appeared in court only rarely since Christmas, had made allegations to the Crown that he had heard of attempts to bribe jurors in the case. With a straight face, Judge K.Y. Dick ordered the Ontario Provincial Police to investigate, and everybody went home.

I complained to the minister of justice, the attorney general, and anyone else who might listen. No one was interested and despite questions in the legislature the silence of Justice triumphed. (After their investigation the police were silent too. No more was heard of the allegations of jury tampering.)

My novel had been accepted by a U.S. publisher in Los Angeles; he wanted me to go on the road and promote it. A sizable royalty advance had accompanied the offer. When school ended, I moved us all out to Costa Mesa, California, and into a lovely home with swimming pool and orange trees in the back yard. It sounded absurd but there appeared a chance that I might make my living as a writer. I started another novel to see if I could repeat the feat.

By fall, any peace and contentment were shattered once again. The FBI in Los Angeles ordered my publisher to visit their offices and answer a few questions concerning one of their authors. They had been told by the Canadian police that I was a front man for PLO terrorists in the States—the novel's subject material—and couldn't possibly have written such a novel because I had no formal education. U.S. immigration asked me to leave the country. And Fred Porter sent a registered letter to say that he'd decided to go with a new trial in Woodstock. Merry Christmas! I flew back to Canada for trial number two, a vastly different affair compared to the first. This time only half the charges were used, the rest held in abeyance as insurance just in case the jury acquitted.

Eric engaged Stewart McKeown under Legal Aid again,

while both I and Guglielmo defended ourselves. Could anything have been more ludicrous than forcing an uneducated and inarticulate Italian immigrant to defend himself in a court of law? Ah, Justice, no wonder you must wear a blindfold.

Although my American publisher offered to pay the enormous fee that Robert Carter wanted in advance to defend me, I knew that for this trial it would be money wasted. On the forty-second day of the charade the jury retired to consider the evidence. . . .

A corridor buzzer sounds. Surprised faces. Cigarettes are butted. Ties straightened. After three days of deliberations they have reached a verdict. Everyone files into court. The defendants stand. The clerk intones: "Jury, look upon the accused. Accused, look upon your jury. How then do you find these defendants on the first charge, guilty or not guilty?"

Time hangs on a thread of silence. My heart skips, flips, bangs against my ribs. The first is the only charge that matters. Conspiracy. All the rest are substantive charges. Window dressing. Without conviction on the first, the rest must fall. The judge explained conspiracy to the jury so that there would be no doubt in anybody's mind what it meant: "Now, if Mr. Foster and Mr. Schwendau were seen together having a cup of coffee, then that's evidence of a conspiracy."

Sure it is.

It is said that a jury's verdict can be anticipated by staring at individual faces. If their eyes hold without wavering, their verdict is for the defense. But if none is prepared to meet a defendant's gaze, then the verdict is guilty. I search vainly. No one will meet my gaze—except Jim Riley, and he is smiling.

"We find the defendants guilty on the first charge."

Thus, with a sick and heavy heart on the fifth day of spring, 1979, I go back to prison.

London, Canada

30 March 1979

Normally there is a three- or four-week gap between conviction and sentencing, during which time, if the crime was nonviolent, the convicted man is given an opportunity to clean up his affairs preparatory to entering prison. Reports are written up for the judge by the Parole Service and the police, giving some idea of the type of sentence to be imposed. Final submissions for probation or suspended sentences are made in court by defense lawyers.

In our case, however, none of this was necessary. Eric and I knew that we'd received the judicial blue plate special. Delays for probation reports or police comments were superfluous, so after conviction we were ordered to return to court the following week for sentencing. Then, without further ado, the three of us were handcuffed quickly and hustled past TV news cameras to a police car for the ride into London's Elgin-Middlesex Counties Detention Center. I was not sorry for the delay. In the United States, time spent in prison before trial and after conviction counts toward time served, but in Canada only jail time served after sentencing starts the Dutch clock to freedom.

Both Eric and Angelo were stunned by the rapidity of events. One moment we were standing in the corridors; minutes later we were manacled and speeding off to prison. Eric was ashen-faced. He had never experienced this sort of thing before. Guglielmo sat looking bewildered.

"What's agonna happen, Fos?" he whispered.

"We're going to jail."

"Jeezkrist!"

Which said it all.

Before leaving court the jury foreman came over and apologized for their verdict. He operated a local engineering and sheet metal company in town.

"A difficult decision, because our hearts were with you completely," he admitted.

"Then you should have followed your hearts."

"Here's my card. If you need a job when you get out of jail, do give me a call. You're a heck of a good salesman."

But apparently not quite good enough for his jury.

The Detention Center on London's outskirts was a sterile maximum-security establishment run for the most part by keen young guards only a few years older than the rowdy teen-aged thugs they were supervising. Upon arrival we were greeted with awe, like some black royalty.

Both guards and inmates had followed our trial with considerable interest on television and in the newspapers. Did we really steal all those millions? How much had we managed to keep for ourselves? Did we need bodyguards? One young tough asked Eric for his mailing address so that he could join our "mob" after release. Another offered to sell me the operational plans for robbing the local Brinks Express office. A steal at five hundred dollars. His girl friend would pick up the money from my lawyer on the outside.

The prison's two-hundred-odd guests were stored in semicircular six- or eleven-man units. Since we were awaiting sentence and considered less of an escape risk than those already sentenced, we were assigned to one of the eleven-man units on the second floor. To move about the building, an incredible series of locked doors had to be negotiated, each one opened by a corridor duty guard lugging enormous keys and a walkie-talkie. A CBer's paradise. Ten-four. I shuddered to think what might happen in case of a serious fire because of this passion for corridor security. Speedy evacuation of the premises would be quite impossible.

Within the living units, eleven rooms opened onto a central day room with uncomfortable plastic tub chairs and square moulded plastic tables where we spent our waking hours, playing cards, reading, or watching television. We also ate our meals there. Except for thirty-minute exercise periods in the gym every other day—outside in a small courtyard if the weather was fine—there was nothing constructive to occupy our mind or body. Although a sizable library and expensively equipped workshop had been installed on the premises, inmates were not permitted to use them. A security officer explained to me rather mysteriously that it all "has to do with security matters." The Armed Forces tenet of keeping men out of mischief by keeping them busy apparently has never dawned on administrators in the penal system in either the States or Canada.

With nothing to do, naturally fistfights and mindless vandalism within units were daily occurrences, both accepted by the staff with an equanimity bordering on indifference. Our rooms were locked during the day lest prisoners be dragged away and beaten out of sight of the duty guard in his glass-enclosed surveillence box. As a result, beatings were administered in the large communal showers attached to the units.

During my previous visit I had not been in residence long enough to realize the Alice in Wonderland quality to the place, certainly not unique in the prison environment. A topsy-turvy logic accompanied every action and reaction, like Newton's Third Law of Motion. Security became the justification for everything, a Hindu deity by which prisoners and staff alike were trapped into its ritualistic performances.

Triweekly strip searches were conducted by tight-lipped, grim-faced guards, although nothing was ever found. Once I asked what they were seeking. "Contraband," I was told—although what constituted contraband was never made clear. Since inmates had no physical contact with anyone except each other, it was difficult to know where such contraband would be obtained or hidden.

An aspirin issue required formal written requests in two copies, followed by the long, complicated door-locking journey to reach an infirmary on the main floor. Normal elapsed time between a request and tablet ingestion took four hours, by which time the headache had long gone or turned into something so powerful that only sleep would soothe it. But if one wanted to stretch out during the day it had to be on the floor to a background noise of TV game shows or soap operas turned on full volume, plus several noisy card games—mostly Hearts. These games and TV channel changing were the fastest route to a punch-out in the shower room between players or viewers who, once matters were settled, returned to their entertainment until the next dispute erupted.

Letters could be written only on lined prison forms and were not to exceed two pages. The reason was censorship, although this was denied hotly by the warden. Pages had to be of uniform size and thickness to fit the Xerox machine, but why copies of inmate correspondence were kept on file was anybody's guess. When in one letter to Helen, who was still in California, I made reference to an inmate complaining how the visiting room had been bugged so that one of his visitor's conversations had been used against him in court, I was ordered to excise the offending three lines.

Later the warden visited me and insisted there were no electronic devices in his visiting rooms, but he refused to read the inmate's recent trial transcript in which the location of the bug had been named by a police officer under oath on the witness stand.

"Then the policeman was lying," the warden exclaimed indignantly.

No doubt.

The prison's well-equipped kitchens were never used to produce meals. Instead, the facilities provided a delivery point for the catering service that held a contract to supply the prison fare. The daily meals arrived on plastic trays in steam carts several hours after preparation, all uniformly ghastly in texture and taste. Not as bad as bologna sandwiches of course.

Eric, who had reached an overweight 236 pounds on his five-foot-six-inch frame during the trial, decided to go on a diet. Our food quality insured his ability to resist temptation. Guglielmo and I shared his food trays.

With nothing to do, under constant worry about the length of sentence to be imposed, and seething with anger at the judicial farce that I had been forced to undergo for five years, I was ripe for a deal on the other charges still outstanding. So, just when the boredom and frustration had become stupefying, Jim Riley turned up for a chat in one of the small interview rooms on the main floor.

He had made a few uncomplimentary remarks to the newspapers about how I wanted to "cut his throat," for which he apologized, claiming he'd been quoted out of context. It was difficult to imagine an alternate context in view of his statement, but I let it slide. He looked very pleased with himself. No wonder.

The deal from the Crown was simplicity itself: I would plead guilty to the more than a dozen outstanding charges and receive one-year concurrent sentences on each. No more jail time. No more trials. Clean slate.

"What about your phony perjury charge? You expect me to plead guilty on that?"

"Everything outstanding."

"No deal."

The interview was over.

The next day an escort took Angelo, Eric, and me back to Woodstock for sentencing. The court was crowded with media, jurymen, and the curious. Stewart McKeown delivered a passionate plea on behalf of Schwendau for a probationary or suspended sentence. Another lawyer spoke for Guglielmo, while I told the judge I didn't believe for one minute he was a clone of Robespierre. We were all wasting words. Misner delivered an amusing presentence lecture for the benefit of the media, then awarded Angie eighteen months in reformatory, Eric and me four years each in penitentiary. Not altogether unexpected.

Fred Porter had the handcuffs removed and invited me into his office for a private conversation. After reconsidering the matter he had decided to drop the perjury charge if I would plead guilty to everything else and use my influence to have Guglielmo do the same. Eric had no further outstanding charges. Additionally, Porter would recommend that I be allowed to take my typewriter and research books with me into prison so that I could continue writing. As a final sweetner he said that he would recommend a minimum-security prison for Eric and myself and early parole.

"You'll be out in sixteen months," he said prophetically.

I told him that I'd consider his offer carefully. Outside the office I was reattached to the other two "criminals," and we returned to London.

The following week the warden visited me, bringing my research books, Olivetti, and 417 pages of plain white bond paper. For some inexplicable security reason every page had a number. I was given a small schoolroom in which to work and, except for meals, allowed to spend my entire waking hours in an orgy of composition. Most of it was thrown out later because it reflected my tattered emotions too closely at the time, but for the remaining weeks of my stay in London I was able to escape into the wonderful world of fantasy and words.

After a week I had to make my decision on the other charges. A not-too-subtle point had been made that, should I elect to go to trial, such a trial could be delayed by the Crown until the four-year sentence had been served. With outstanding charges pending, there would of course be no opportunity for parole and every likelihood that the Crown would break up the remaining charges and take them to trial one at a time.

It had also been made clear that I could spend the rest of my life going from court to prison and back again, never managing to get myself cleared.

These "arguments" were mighty persuasive. I capitulated.

Five weeks slipped past during which I completed my book and the formality of appeal on my conviction, the latter a waste of time without benefit of representative counsel on the outside.

For our first weeks after sentencing Eric and Angie tried frantically to arrange release on appeal bonds. Gradually the idea of facing the inevitable became less distasteful and they spoke less and less about appealing. Both suffered the initial shock that I had experienced in Terminal Island when, like a fish hooked firmly on the line, the first reaction is to wriggle like hell. During those first weeks in California's prison system my hands and feet had broken out in hundreds of water blisters, a nervous reaction brought about by the tremendous psychological stresses I was undergoing. Headaches, panic, claustrophobia, are all part of it.

There can be nothing more stressful to an active person than enforced inactivity with no means of physical escape. Relief comes only by disciplining the body to accept its new circumstances while allowing the mind to follow whatever will-o'-the-wisp it wishes to pursue. The whole being must be turned inward until, as any good Buddhist knows, time no longer matters because it doesn't exist.

A week later Guglielmo was snatched out of the unit late one night for shipment to Guelph Reformatory. On the evening of May 2, 1979, Eric and I were brought down to the maximum-security units pending arrival of transport to take us to Kingston Penitentiary in the morning. It was all very cloak-and-dagger.

Our prison garb was exchanged for our street clothing, all personal possessions were returned, checked off, then packed in yellow duffel bags. My typewriter in its carrying case received a special FRAGILE label. To avoid any suicide attempts, our belts and shoes were left outside the cells before lock up. Two other pairs of shoes and belts lay in front of adjacent doors in the unit. We would not be traveling alone to Kingston, but the identity of our companions remained unknown until morning because the guards refused to divulge their names for "security reasons."

Great secrecy surrounded these movements between prisons. There was a fear that outside confederates might discover the schedule and decide to bushwhack the vehicle. It was patently absurd, but over the years authorities had convinced themselves that this was a real and ever-present danger. Yet no convict I met in Canada or the United States ever suggested anything as foolish as hijacking one of those prison buses. Escape plans provided always for a singular—sometimes dual—departure, undetected and when least suspected, preferably at night. Taking out a crowded bus along a busy highway in broad daylight was not the answer. But bureaucratic fantasies run deep.

After breakfast we were placed in the holding tank and got to meet our companions, a squeamish child molester who spoke in grunts and refused to look anyone in the eye, and a personable young lad just sentenced to eight years for manslaughter. He had caught his wife *in flagrante delicto* with a local Chinaman and blown both away with a shotgun. His trial had been almost as sensational locally as ours, although with a much stiffer penalty.

Midmorning our bus arrived from Windsor and Chatham with a group of sleepy transportees already on board. Eric and I were handcuffed and shackled together with short ankle chains, making it impossible for us to walk without careful mutual coordination. Our duffel bags were loaded in the rear and we were escorted cautiously down the aisle to an empty double seat. Donny—I shall call him Donny—and the child molester took their places across the aisle. The other passengers gave us incurious stares and remained silent. Guard and driver came aboard and we backed out of the garage past the electric overhead doors.

Huzzah! We were on our way to the Big House.

Gray skies wept outside the windows with suitable sentiment. Tires whined on the slick pavement. Inside the atmosphere was laden with cigarette smoke, sour, sweating bodies, and tiny prisms of uncertainty that drifted among the riders like dust motes.

Donny leaned across to inquire if either Eric or I had been to KayPee, as Kingston Pen was known among the cognoscenti. I admitted to driving past once or twice and flying over it many times, but never being inside. He wondered a little fearfully what it was going to be like.

A laconic coffee-colored black from Chatham turned slightly in his seat and observed softly: "It's a drag, man, but a whole heap better'n any one of these goddamn provincial joints. At least in the pen a man's got his freedom with none of that chickenshit you gotta put up with in these local buckets. Keep cool, kid. The time will float by."

We began to talk. Jesse had been in all the worst places across the country during his twenty years of prison time for bank robberies.

"Y'see, the law says if you get two years or better you gotta go to the pen. Under two years means provincial reformatory. So anyone with two years less a day is carrying heavy jail time so far as these provincial buckets are concerned. High-risk dudes. Shackles, chains, round-the-clock surveillence, right? But at the pen if you ain't doin' ten years or better, you're considered to be doin' small time, right? Things is real easy at the pen for low timers. How big a bit you got, kid?"

When Donny told him eight years Jesse laughed.

"Sheet, you got it whupped. You'll be out in under three years. I'd take book on it. You can do it standing on your head."

During late afternoon, after several stops along the way to pick up passengers, we arrived at the East Toronto Detention Center to spend the night. Eric and I shared a room and a double bunk.

Prison regulations specified single-bed rooms or cells for all prisoners, but the Toronto facility was so overcrowded that two men bunking in quarters designed for one person had become the norm.

By nightfall our unit on the fifth floor had been filled with arrivals from northern parts of the province plus a few shipped from several of the Kingston penitentiaries who had been out attending Toronto courts. They were young men for the most part, with tattoo-covered muscles, cautious eyes, and a studied indifference to the guards and the surroundings. Everyone smoked nervously and played cards or talked in low tones. Conspiracy lurked everywhere.

A much bigger bus collected us all the next morning. The Blue Goose, as it was known, took us nonstop to Millhaven Penitentiary. A half-dozen of the toughest prisoners clanked down the aisle with heavy footsteps to the accompanied murmurs from the other passengers of "Take it cool, y'hear?" and "Good luck."

Except for the outside perimeter of guard towers and the double row of high razor-wire fencing, the place looked no different from the London Detention Center. But inside, things were vastly different. Just the sight of the infamous Millhaven was sufficient to subdue everyone on board the bus. The brutality and hopeless conditions beyond the wire were known intimately by several of those still with us. As we drove out one of them explained: "Like it's this way, see. If they figure you're a wise guy who's never going to get his act together, they check you into the Special Handling Unit. That's endsville, see. Cells are like steel boxes. Twenty hours a day lockup—longer if they decide to make you really squirm. Some guys never get out. No parole. No release. When you hit the Special Handling Unit it's all over because there's no way back, see. They go nuts in there. Too hard to handle then. There's no way they can let anyone out again. They kill them. Living death in a steel drum. Me, I'd rather be dead for real instead of doing it their way. The rotten fuckers!"

Five more left us at Collins Bay. They appeared delighted at the prospect of returning home after their weeks of court sittings in Toronto. From the stifling security and miserable conditions of Toronto's prison, they were returning to the comfort and easy familiarity of their peer group. Home is where the heart is. Our next stop was KayPee.

Kingston Penitentiary was built in the early part of the last century as a military barracks for British Army regulars who had been posted along the north shore of Lake Ontario to guard against American adventurism. Change-over from barracks to penal institution came later.

A date of 1833 appears on a stone facing above the archway into the central prison dome, so it is reasonable to assume that by then a change was already under way. During those early years citizens drove out from Kingston town by horse and buggy on Sunday afternoons to take pot shots at the convicts with bows and arrows from the safety of the walls. Whether this was by private invitation of the prison's governor or merely accepted Sunday afternoon sport for the locals, history doesn't make clear.

With the passage of time the city of Kingston grew until the prison, its quaint stone church, guards' homes, and vast farmlands were swallowed in the gulp of urban thirst for space. Today the penitentiary is practically downtown.

The Blue Goose pulled up in front of the main entrance, a narrow stone sally port built to accommodate horse-drawn carriages. Our chains and handcuffs were removed by brown-uniformed guards and we were marched inside the walls to Reception for processing, with our duffel bags bringing up the rear.

Although the day had turned sunny and cool with a fresh wind blowing in from the lake, the prison compound wore the drab gray uniform of time. Buildings that had weathered at least eight generations of men's miseries stood in granite Victorian hauteur as a challenge to the bleeding heart of change. Each window façade seemed to be sneering in derision at the latest group of arrivals—new "fish," in the vernacular.

At the back of the compound lay the prison's yard and playing field, enclosed on three sides by massive walls and guard towers. Behind the rear wall, hidden from sight, lapped the waters of Lake Ontario. So close. The playing field had been seeded for 150 years with cinders from the coal-fired central furnaces. So high had the ground level been raised above the soil that the only flowers that grew were dandelions. It was a dreary place filled with ghosts and bitter sorrows. I could feel its past like a living presence everywhere I turned.

After bedding and clothing issue, cold shower, and mug shots we were escorted along a narrow roadway beside the west wall and around a corner into the range block for cell assignments. Before the riot of 1963 this central block held over six hundred men on four levels. After riot repairs, the top two levels were closed off with a false ceiling and the prison population lowered to under three hundred. An extensive modernization program had been under way for several years in an attempt to produce an acceptable slice of Canadiana from this monstrous Victorian anachronism.

KayPee's function had changed too. It became a haven for prisoners in protective custody: child molesters, rapists, stool pigeons, and convicted cops who had to be segregated from the regular prison populations for fear of summary retribution by other inmates. On the east side of the complex a psychiatric center operated for the mentally deranged. But KayPee had become a regional reception center where the newly convicted were assessed, interviewed, tested, and examined over a six-week period prior to shipment to other neighborhood prisons.

After collecting a blanket, pillow, and toilet brush issue from a duty guard in the central dome, I was conducted to G Range and given a cell on the main floor. Eric drew one on the second level, which meant that he had to climb steel stairs and use the catwalk to reach his new home. The cells were small, brightly painted over the cracked plaster, and quite comfortable. Each had a writing desk, sink, toilet, and—unlike the provincial jails—well-stuffed mattress and spring bed. Lighting was ample for reading. New fish were issued a set of earphones for listening to any of the five local radio stations piped into the cells.

I sat down on the bed to contemplate my new surroundings. The ground-floor cells opened onto a wide day-room corridor that provided two television sets and numerous wooden chairs and tables for card games, backgammon, monopoly, or whatever amusement was available from the recreation department. The second-level catwalk overlooked this day room and residents on the second floor shared the space. Since there were thirty cells on each level the day-room corridor must have been terribly overcrowded in the days when all four levels were used for housing prisoners.

I was not unhappy with my condition. In Latin America I had lived in much worse hotels and paid gladly for the privilege because that's all that was available. Without doubt a good percentage of the world's population would give their eyeteeth to be awarded such generous individual accommodation. I decided that prison punishment was all a matter of personal perspective, and thanked my lucky stars for the freedom of a penitentiary in which to serve time instead of the suffocating atmosphere of a provincial prison.

Supper came early at four o'clock. In sequence the ranges emptied to join a swift-moving line past the kitchen delivery windows where food trays were filled, mugs charged with milk, tea, or coffee, and everything taken back to the cells to be eaten. Food quality was excellent, but there were no seconds. I decided that there had to be a place for me in the kitchens.

Both Eric and I opted to waive the IQ, psychological, and mechanical testing, which would cut our stay at KayPee in half. Neither of us was interested in learning a prison trade, life skills, or discovering that we were latent psychopaths. In any case, after the age of forty-five every man is irredeemable and well past salvation.

To pass the time Eric, still keeping to his diet and delivering a sizable portion of every food tray to me, took up jogging during the two-hour exercise period each afternoon. He looked ridiculous huffing around the cindered perimeter beside the walls. For a while I joined him for the exercise. But after a single lap I began to develop chest pains and an alarming shortness of breath and had to stop and rest. Angina pectoris never crossed my mind.

"Too many cigarettes," he'd yell gleefully and continue pounding the cinders relentlessly.

By our third week he could run nonstop for thirty minutes and had managed to shed nearly thirty pounds since the day of our verdict. His goal was to reach 140 pounds and run ten miles before release. In the end it took him only seven months to accomplish it.

In my second week I went to work in the kitchens preparing desserts for the staff dining room and helping serve on the food line. Working in kitchen whites provided an opportunity to get the best food, the choicest steaks, and freshest fruit in nearly unlimited quantities. Blocks of cheese, sliced meats, and pastries could be spirited back to the range and either given to friends or traded with strangers for goodies from the prison commissary. Within the limits imposed by my surroundings, I wanted for nothing.

Those in protective custody lived in D Range and took their meals at the delivery windows only after the other ranges had been locked down. Daily I watched these unfortunates pass along the serving line, prisoners in a prison within a prison.

Finally, when they were all through, guards brought down the three men living in exiled isolation cells on the third level. They had been hidden away since their conviction for the sex slaying of a Portuguese shoeshine boy in Toronto. So revolting was their crime that not even the normal sanctuary of protective custody was sufficient to save them from attack. They had twenty-four more years to wait before any parole consideration. Old men by then.

When they entered the line, kitchen guards stepped closer to the servers, making certain that no one spit on the food trays or slipped a carving knife through the opening into someone's belly. Casual chatter ceased. Hostility lay in every serving. The trio moved slowly, like somnambulents, their faces fixed in masks of indifference. But their eyes were their most arresting feature. They were all quite dead.

Except for one hare-brained drive to Woodstock in the back of a police car at three o'clock in the morning for a three-minute court appearance and a return to Kingston the same day, my time passed uneventfully. I wrote letters, read a great deal, and delivered vast amounts of illicit food to the men on my range. On the last day of May I was transferred to Joyceville.

The day of the move turned out to be one of those typically balmy spring mornings when it is difficult to imagine a time when man and nature were not in harmony. From the barred open windows of the bus sensuous smells of earth, manure, and growing things came wafting in to titillate the passengers. There was a sense of relief to be leaving KayPee. Eric was left behind. He had made himself much too useful as clerk in the Reception office to be transferred. He looked very glum when I waved good-by.

Joe, my chained seat mate, sniffed the air contentedly.

"Smell that. Freedom, that's what that is, by God!"

I didn't disagree. We had worked in the kitchen together. He had a fast, acerbic wit that I enjoyed. A man who drifted through life with one eyebrow cocked in perpetual skepticism while laughing at the human comedy. At one time he'd been news editor with one of the nation's leading publishing groups, but instead of sticking to scribing the news, he'd decided to branch out into bank robbery on the theory that his job and background made him the least likely suspect in a police investigation. He was wrong. The judge gave him ten years for this aberration of personality. He had been paroled but returned to prison for leaving the country to attend a golf tournament without permission from his parole officer. He wasn't bitter, merely cynical about the turn of events.

"Once you've got a record, my friend, you are a nonperson. That old SIN number that's supposed to be such a secret turns up everywhere to tattle on you. You become unemployable, unwanted, and unloved. So I went to Florida to play in a tournament. What was my crime? Answer me that?"

I couldn't.

Neither apparently could the Parole Board because within three months of our bus ride he was released. But his business, family, and future had already been destroyed by an unsympathetic parole officer.

Joyceville Penitentiary had been built after World War II to take the overflow from Collins Bay and Kingston. Situated on the edge of the Rideau River and canal system twenty miles north of Kingston, it was considered a medium-security prison for older men—older being defined as anyone past twenty-seven. Youthful offenders were sent to the gladiator school at Collins Bay where they could test their mettle among members of their peer group.

Joyceville housed 450 prisoners at capacity but was seldom full. Outwardly it looked more like a military barracks than a prison. Four-story living units enclosed a rectangular parade square on three sides. A fourth side housed administration offices, chapel, staff dining room, gymnasium, library, exercise room, hobby shop, and infirmary. At the back, huge lawns sloped down to the river.

Superficially, at least, its relatively modern construction, greenery, and pastoral view of the river with scattered tree-canopied farms beyond was not unlike Terminal Island prison with its delightful ocean setting. But any resemblance ended there. At T.I. prisoners slept in 150-man dormitories on double bunks and used communal washrooms. In Joyceville every man had his own comfortable six-by-nine-foot room with solid door, window view, desk, basin, and toilet with proper seat. Radios, pictures, pinups, and hobby crafts were allowed in the rooms. When the door closed, there was a luxurious sense of total privacy. This personal privacy is the single greatest difference between the Canadian and U.S. prison systems.

Once past the electric steel mesh gates we were unshackled and, lugging our personal possessions, led into the Reception area to be introduced to "Clipboard Bill." Bill Buculla's job was to provide stewardship over every new arrival for his first two weeks. He led a guided tour of indoctrination to show and explain how the prison operated. A decent, sympathetic man, he wandered the premises like a penal Vanderdecken with his clipboard of names, always with a half-dozen new fish in tow, helping, advising, listening politely to complaints. He should have entered the priesthood. He might have become a saint.

Clipboard Bill handed out room assignments. I drew number 28 in D Block on the first floor. It overlooked the main parade square. Rooms with forest or river view were at a premium and awarded on the basis of seniority. I didn't anticipate being around the place long enough to qualify.

Meals were delivered from the central kitchens by food trolleys into the unit day rooms located at the end of each floor. These day rooms provided cafeteria-style tables for eating and, after meals, a restful place for card games or watching color television. A bottomless coffee and a fresh milk urn were always on tap and, in addition, a lovely fully stocked refrigerator should anyone feel peckish between meals. The food was excellent, the atmosphere relaxed and congenial, and everyone encouraged to develop their own interest. What more could anyone ask for— except freedom?

I unpacked my Olivetti and set to work, something I had been unable to do at KayPee because of the noise from the open barred cells. In Joyceville, with my door closed, I could work at all hours without fear of disturbing anyone.

At the end of two weeks' touring with Clipboard Bill, I asked to work in the library. Everyone had to have a work assignment, although most employment was created to give inmates the illusion of doing something constructive. The prison ran a well-paying industrial complex, producing sheet metal products for use by the federal government, but there was a long waiting list for such choice earning spots at the industry shops and kitchens.

Rudi Mier operated the prison library. A cautious Dutchman with a kindly nature, he accepted me as an assistant librarian even though he had four prisoners assisting already.

On the first day it was clear that he expected nothing from me but to keep out of mischief. He gave me permission to lug my Olivetti to and from "work," along with various files that I needed, and I selected a secluded table on which to work next to the latest editions of the *Encyclopaedia Britannica*. Talk about having reference material at my fingertips. The spring days passed swiftly in a delight of self-indulgent prose.

Late in June Jim Riley turned up, not unexpectedly, bubbling with good humor and the milk of human kindness, to take me back to Woodstock for the finale. Unmarked police car, a stop for milkshake and hamburgers along the way, smiles and chuckles throughout. Did I still intend to plead guilty on the remaining charges, he wondered?

"I'll plead guilty—except for the perjury charge."

He beamed. "No sweat. We're in business. You might think about dropping your appeal, too. Parole applications are harder when you've an appeal outstanding."

Later that afternoon in court, Guglielmo and I did as we had agreed earlier in the judge's chambers. Another judge had been sent from Owen Sound to hear the pleas because Judge Dick had excused himself from hearing anything on our case. I couldn't blame the poor man.

Fred Porter kept his word, too. Guglielmo was released shortly thereafter to return home on a work-release parole program, while a few weeks later, after dropping my appeal, I was transferred to the minimum-security camp at Frontenac. Finally things were beginning to look up.

For one last time I wore handcuffs and leg irons. I arrived on a warm sunny August day when trees and birds and life were dozing after their peak of growth. At Frontenac, lush gardens circled the lawns and walkways. From the back lawn I had an unobstructed and beautific view of open fields, ripening wheat, yellowing hay. Cows stood munching contentedly, flicking flies, feeling the sun's warmth on their dappled hides. Every fence in sight had an exit through an unlocked gate. And there was a new smell. A different smell. More powerful than the earth or animals or fresh breezes coming off the lake. For an instant it watered my eyes, blurring the splendid sight that lay before me. It was the smell of freedom. With a shock I remembered that it was my birthday.

The cuffs and chains were unlocked. My escort drove away. In the lobby I found a pay phone and called Helen in California telling her to pack the suitcases and children into the car and head for Kingston. The end of our ordeal was in sight.

Or so I thought at the time ...

Kingston, Canada

25 March 1980

At four o'clock in the morning the angina pains come back without warning. I have just returned from the bathroom at the end of the corridor of cubicles. When I climb into bed the pain starts. Very lightly. A mere caress, as though chiding me for the presumption in believing it would never return.

I lie still in silent disbelief. So soon? The pain grows, spreading into my shoulder; the left, where it had gone before my heart attack. I fumble for a nitro pill and lay it beneath my tongue. In two minutes or less the angina retreats to wherever it has been hiding these past two months.

As the pain departs on the wings of nitroglycerin it becomes possible to persuade myself that all is well. Rationalizing, I pretend it wasn't angina. Not really. Something much simpler. A pulled muscle perhaps? Brought about by an awkward sleeping position, so that when I climbed out of bed a chain of internal muscular contractions resulted in what felt exactly like angina but actually wasn't. Mind power. I fall asleep.

At 4:30 A.M. the duty guard awakens the man in the next cubicle. Bobby-Barrel-Belly works the milk separator in the prison farm's dairy. The job is a soft touch but the hours are terrible unless you like meeting the dawn.

I listen to Bobby dress, vaguely aware that the angina is with me. Ridiculous. What have I been doing wrong? I've followed the doctor's advice exactly: short walks, increasing gradually in tempo and distance until I'm walking two miles daily without tiring or discomfort. I have lifted nothing heavier than ten pounds and taken a one-hour nap every afternoon. During the last visit to the hospital's Out-Patient Clinic the doctor pronounced me fully recovered and able to resume normal working activities. Now I have angina. What went wrong?

This terrible realization frightens me. Somewhere along my coronary arteries there is another restriction forming to hold back the blood that is needed to feed my heart muscle. But is the blockage at a critical juncture or only a small tributary? Will it kill me and if so, when?

Fingers of panic clutch my heart to set it hammering—as much as is possible for it to hammer with the daily Inderal doses I've been taking. The pain hardens. I fumble for another nitro, knocking the bottle on the floor. Quickly I scramble from bed and begin a flat-palmed grope to find it. Bobby-Barrel-Belly frames the open doorway beneath the dim nightlight.

"You all right?" he whispers.

He is my age and finishing a ten-year sentence for kidnapping a tractor-trailer and its driver. Once he was a sergeant in the paratroops. Tough as nails. Now he's overweight, flabby-faced, and wearing his graying hair in an outdated wethead pompadour. Back in December when I was going through hell during the prelude to my heart attack, he heard me groan and sob in the small hours and, unasked, came in to sit on the bed with an arm around my shoulders to comfort me. Silly really. The helpful and helpless in the blindness of the night. Yet I appreciated the gesture because it came from his heart.

He likes telling anyone who will listen that if his crime had happened in Quebec, the driver a British Trade Commissioner, and he'd forced the federal government into providing him with an airplane to Cuban exile, his sentence would have been two years with parole in eight months. Unfortunately he chose a truck with Ontario plates.

I explain my problem and he joins me on the floor, neither of us prepared to turn on the bedside lamp and risk disturbing the other sleeping men. The cubicles have no doors, no top or bottom to the walls, and were designed for cheap partial privacy. Every cough, sneeze, belch, and fart echoes throughout the high-ceilinged dormitory among the forty cubicles. Originally the place served as a garage for Collins Bay until someone got the bright idea of turning it into a minimum-security camp outside the prison walls. The second-floor dorms house eighty men, but the place is never filled to capacity. Releases, escapes, returns to maximum security for disciplinary infractions, all take their toll every week. Frontenac's population is highly transitory.

My chest pain is quite frightful now, made worse by hunching over and scrambling about the floor.

"Got it!" Bobby exclaims hoarsely.

I grab the bottle gratefully and extract one tiny white magic tablet. Bobby watches in the vague light.

"You gonna be okay now?"

"Sure, fine. Thanks."

He nods and departs while I sit on the edge of the bed and feel the tablet soothe away the raging pain. No doubt what it is. No point trying to kid myself. Face the music. The problem is irreversible, like the tide. My regimen of physical activities and medical supplements has accomplished nothing. The doctors lied. Hope spooned to another anxious and gullible patient to prevent the hysteria and stress that come from being forced to face the terrible truth. The boogeyman will get you if you don't watch out! Hello, boogeyman.

There is a theory, first advanced by Dr. Hans Selye, University of Montreal, that stress is the root cause of all human disease and cardiovascular disabilities. Dr. Arthur Gladman, medical director of the Everett A. Gladman Memorial Hospital in Oakland, California, stated flatly: "I'm convinced that every disease from the common cold to cancer is a product of stress and its effect on our immune system."

Stress, it appears, can make you sick in the way it affects the body's immune systems. Under stress the white cells of the immune system alter, allowing sickness to set in. In situations of acute danger or threat, the body pours out hormones that provide additional strength in order to fight the challenge or flee the danger. In primitive times this was a useful asset. Civilized society won't allow us to fight and we can't run away from our problems, so the extra energy isn't used and remains in the body to weaken the immune system. Stress-triggered disease then attacks the weakest parts of the body. This varies from person to person. With smokers the attack can come in the lungs or the throat; for high-powered salesmen and business executives it can mean heart attacks.

The theory assumes that most of us enter the world as tiny perfect beings. Whatever good or bad genes we've inherited are with us throughout life. Traits such as baldness, visual acuity, physique, facial characteristics, and even longevity are products of our DNA heritage. But emotionally, after age eighteen, we're on our own. We make our own emotional beds and sleep in them by our own choosing.

Those colds we shrugged off in youth have, by midlife, become debilitating forces that put us in bed several days. By old age they are killers. Since my coronary I have consumed dozens of books covering these worries. My appetite for medical and physical knowledge is insatiable. I haven't been this interested in my body since puberty. If I'm to fall apart, as eventually I must under the immutable laws of nature, then I'd like to learn as much as possible on how the process can be slowed. Instead of racing headlong off the precipice of self-destruction, I'd prefer to tackle the matter at a more leisurely and perhaps reflective pace. After all, in the final analysis, what the hell is the rush?

Startling information can be found on the shelves of any local lending library. For example: most of mankind's major illnesses have been described in medical publications since Hippocrates. Coronary disease is never mentioned. "Ah," you say, "but in ancient times people never lived long enough to develop such maladies." Quite true. When men in their thirties were considered bordering on dotage and children's survival rates from birth to age nine were less than 15 percent, bodies had little time to develop arteriosclerosis.

Yet even as late as 1920 coronary disease was relatively uncommon in North America. The late Dr. Paul Dudley White, President Eisenhower's coronary physician, recalled that in the first two years after setting up his practice in 1921 he saw only two or three coronary cases. The coronary is a twentieth-century phenomenon.

Diet, exercise, family history, cholesterol levels in the

blood, are important factors in the development of heart disease and many other illnesses. Although medical opinions vary on the body's ability to provide a necessary level of antibodies to combat disease, there is one point on which opinions are unanimous. Stress is a killer. Volumes of published evidence prove it.

Among animals, only man has the ability to perceive time. Today, time moves unrelentingly faster and faster, forcing man to compete, first with himself, then against everyone else. Such competitiveness has brought about disastrous consequences for man in modern society. During the Victorian era people ate virtually the same things that we do today, they exercised less and weighed considerably more, but they didn't have as much heart disease. Why? Because they did not lead the stressful lives of today's competitive society.

Sir William Osler, the Canadian physician and scholar, wrote extensively about his observations of angina patients during the early years of this century. Although he did not live long enough to view the epidemic proportions to which the coronary phenomenon grew, he drew very shrewd conclusions about the classic angina-prone type. He wrote: "It is not the delicate neurotic person who is prone to angina, but the robust, the vigorous in mind and body, the keen and ambitious man, the indicator of whose engine is always at 'full speed ahead' ... the well-set man of from forty-five to fifty-five years of age, with military bearing, iron gray hair, and florid complexion."

Except for the florid complexion, Osler's 1897 treatise "On Angina Pectoris and Allied States" might have been describing me. What he is saying quite simply is that life in the fast lane creates stress and stress can cause angina.

During the 1930s when I came into this world, mortality from coronaries in North America increased by more than an astounding 100 percent in one four-year period. People couldn't cope with events, couldn't adjust to the destruction of their lives by forces over which they had no control and didn't understand. The loss of pride, the misery and degradation of soup kitchens, massive unemployment, all brought millions to the brink of despair. Heart attacks became almost a method of involuntary self-destruction.

In World War II at the Battle of Stalingrad, Russian soldiers fell back block by block, stubbornly resisting the German Army's attempts to conquer their city. The battle lasted three years, much of it a result of hand-to-hand combat and under constant emotional stress. The effects were catastrophic. During 1942 and 1943 hypertension rates provided by Russian medical records indicated an increase from 4.1 percent to 64 percent of the population. Worst of all, few of those who managed to survive returned to normal health when hostilities ended. By the early Sixties, most had died, long before reaching old age.

In recent times a report by Dr. Thomas Holmes of Seattle's University of Washington to the American Association for the Advancement of Science produced evidence to show that any great change—either good or bad—produces stress. Dr. Holmes devised a scale assigning point values to changes affecting test subjects.

If the score totaled more than 300 in a given year, individuals could be in for serious physical problems. In his survey, 80 percent of those exceeding 300 became pathologically depressed, had heart attacks, or developed serious ailments.

Below the 300 score, problems fell away dramatically. Yet even a score of 150 was sufficient to affect 33 percent of those tested. The Holmes chart, reproduced here in part, gives some idea on how his rating system worked.

Event	Value
Death of a spouse	100
Divorce	73
Marital separation	65
Jail term	63
Love affair	63
Personal injury or illness	53
Marriage	50
Fired from job	47
Marital reconciliation	45
Retirement	45

Even such mundane events as a vacation, change in residence, or a son and daughter leaving home were considered stressful.

Tabulating events in my life for the preceding year, I produced a horrifying score of 462. No wonder I had a heart attack and now, two months later, the first stirrings of another. Something had gone wrong with the medical prognostications. Is the mighty Lord Koval merely a mortal after all? What am I to do? Where is the comfort and solace I need, the advice to guide me along the paths of longevity and righteousness? Certainly not within the Canadian penitentiary system.

Dr. Ted DeJager visits Frontenac for sick call once a week. There are formalities to be observed in order to have one's name posted for his examination. Hours are from 7:30 to 8:00 A.M. It doesn't pay to be late or DeJager locks the door and leaves, telling whoever is left to come back next week for diagnosis. Since my heart attack I need no longer go through the formalities of procedure and can drop in at the end of the line.

There are the usual ten or twelve men waiting for him when I come down from the dormitory. Their ailments are both real and imaginary, most stemming from the farm and dairy work. Cuts, sprains, bruises, and those who simply want a couple of days off from the tedium of seven-day work weeks in the huge barns, cleaning and milking eighty head of cattle. During winter the animals are penned, so it's a thankless, filthy job.

Yet everyone must serve an apprenticeship either on the farm or in the barns, doing heavy bullwork before being permitted to move on to more leisurely and less regimented chores. My first six weeks the previous August and September were spent as a farm laborer bringing in hay and clearing stones from the erupting landscape. Then I moved indoors to become the camp's baker and pastry chef. My puff pastries, cream-filled swans, succulent napoleons, and aromatic sticky buns became legendary.

DeJager listens carefully to my new angina problem.

"Any pains now?"

I shake my head. He taps the end of his pen against his front teeth. An annoying distraction.

"But they'll come back again tonight, I'd be willing to bet. Leave it with me. I'll try and arrange an appointment with Gary Burggraf. He's a cardiologist."

"So is Dr. Koval."

"Yes, but I'd rather have Burggraf see you to make the final decision."

"What final decision?"

"Whether you should have a by-pass operation."

"Ah!"

He snaps his bag closed with a theatrical flourish, like an itinerant magician at the end of his magic show. "Leave all the arrangements to me. If you need to have a by-pass operation, then I'll see that you get one."

He makes it sound like a threat . . . almost.

I'm not impressed, finding it difficult now to believe anything he might say after treating me for indigestion instead of acute angina this past December. At least now when I say that I have angina he doesn't argue. Progress is all a matter of perspective.

The male nurse from Collins Bay Penitentiary who accompanied Ted stacks away the inmate medical records. As the morning work buzzer sounds in the outside hall, nurse and doctor depart through the side door to DeJager's car. The highly polished Mercedes sedan is a source of weekly envy for both staff and inmates, who dislike his ostentation.

Standing at the window in the medical room, I watch them drive off. Except for weekly visits to the doctor, the medical room is off limits to inmates. I'm the exception. There are actually three rooms: a small reception area, a toilet, and a tiny office with an enormous blond oak desk. Once DeJager leaves, the place becomes my private hideaway.

When I returned from hospital after the heart attack with orders to do no physical work for two months, the prison director, Jim Caird, offered me these premises so that I could work on my book. He's a likable no-nonsense sort of individual with hound-dog features and hooded eyes that don't quite conceal his amusement at the world in general. Caird is a professional trouble-shooter, the type of man that corporate directors send in to clean up those horrible fiscal, administrative, or personnel messes left by politicians and their incompetent sycophants. A man to respect. I accepted his offer and spent weeks in happy seclusion, surrounded by my research files, reference books, radio, and typewriter.

My first-floor window looks out on the parking lot where Helen and the children park when they come to visit every weekday after supper. Running the length of this parking area is a long, low building housing the penitentiary system's stores. In the military it would be called the Quartermaster's Stores. Every consumable item used by the regional penitentiaries passes through here.

Regional Stores are operated by a half-dozen convicts from Frontenac and similar number of females from the Women's Penitentiary in town, the latter bussed in and out from work. On-the-job fraternization is discouraged under threat of return to maximum security, but these threats are made in vain because when sexually starved men and women are placed in close proximity, coupling is inevitable regardless of consequence.

A narrow paved road loops from the parking lot, around the end of Regional Stores, to join the circumferential roadway of Collins Bay Penitentiary. The southeast guard tower is within hailing distance of my window. Freedom is so near and yet so far. Frontenac's prisoners are just as imprisoned as those on the other side of the high stone wall. Here, the amenities are better. That's the only difference.

I pull my portable Olivetti from under the desk and reel in a blank sheet of paper. The second novel is nearly complete. Only that surge before the climax remains before it's finished. The point where all the loose threads are gathered. Then the ending. No problem with the ending. I have that mapped out in my mind already. A zinger, to leave the reader satisfied. The blank page stares up at me.

Nothing comes to my fingers. No clever words, no succinct

phrase to frame a scattered thought. My brain is as blank as the page. Hesitantly I peck out B Y - P A S S with one finger and study the letters with a degree of curiosity.

A few weeks ago on the television program "60 Minutes" I saw a segment on the history of a man who had undergone by-pass surgery. A young man. Much younger than I. The cameras entered the operating theater and observed the operation's highlights: the yawning chest cavity cranked open at the breast by two stainless-steel clamps, the purple-red heart muscle pulsating angrily within its Saran-wrap casing, the coronary arteries clearly visible.

First, blood circulation was by-passed through a heart-lung machine to give the body's dharma a chance to rest. The heart quivered to a stop and lay twitching like some high-priced thoroughbred scratched from the race at the starting gate. A yard of vein was removed from the patient's leg and snipped neatly into usable lengths, then each strip was sutured carefully from the massive aorta at the top of the heart onto one coronary artery, just ahead of the blockage. Three times the process was repeated. A magnifying glass was used to check the stitches afterward to make certain the connections were seated smoothly and secure enough to withstand the surge of blood pressure when the machine was disconnected. A three-hour operation crammed into fifteen minutes.

Finally, the critical restarting of the heart. For at least two hours it had remained dormant, bathed in a salty solution of nutrients designed to keep the electrical circuits within the muscle alert and healthy. Slowly, ever so slowly, blood and air were returned to the heart and lungs. At first nothing happened. Then a perceptible tremble began to convulse the organ. Electrical circuitry from the brain started taking over. The beat returned. Life would continue, for a while at least.

In the last clips of film the patient was shown playing Little League ball with his children a year after his operation. He looked strong and healthy, happy to be alive and refereeing the ball game. A uniformed runner from third base slid to home plate as the catcher scooped the ball. "Safe!" the referee yelled.

It was a slick Hollywood-style presentation that left no doubt in the viewer's mind that open-heart surgery, whether for coronary by-passes, valve replacements, or transplants, was now almost on a par with tonsillectomy or appendectomy. It convinced me. At least until I discussed the subject with a young intern during my last checkup at Hotel Dieu Hospital.

One of Koval's initiates, he hadn't seen the television program. In fact he admitted that it had been weeks since he'd had time to stop long enough to listen to the radio or read a newspaper. But he knew enough about open-heart surgery to scare the wits out of me when I inquired. He paused before answering to recheck my file folder to make certain I wasn't slated for out-patient surgery.

"You're not thinking of having a by-pass, are you?"

"Of course not. Merely curious. Have you ever seen the operation performed?"

"Twice. I assisted, supposedly. 'Stand well back from the table, doctor'—you know the type of treatment given to a new boy. But I did see the entire procedure. Interesting. We don't do any of them here. Kingston General has all the facilities."

"What happened to the patients?"

"One lived, the other died."

He gave his brown cowlick a quick flip off the forehead and removed his glasses. The lenses were thick. His eyes appeared to shrink without them. He massaged the bridge of his nose, eyes shut.

"Older men, I suppose—the patients?"

"Your age. The one who died was under forty."

"Jezuz."

He delivered a short tutorial nod to precede this advice: "If the choice was mine, I'd opt for the medication route. Just as effective and one hell of a lot safer than invasive surgery. You don't get to hear too much about the failures. Only the successes."

"What goes wrong?"

"A hundred different things. You've heard the term 'postoperative complications'?"

I nodded. He replaced his glasses, enlarging his eyes.

"It's a surgical catch-all to cover every contingency. But the bottom line is that the patient dies. There are lots of postoperative complications with open-heart surgery. When it works, it's a Godsend—when it works. Be thankful you don't need it."

I put on my shirt and went out to find the escort for the trip back to Frontenac, no doubt in my mind that if put to the test of choosing between surgery and pills, I'd opt for the pills.

But that was two weeks ago when the angina was still a fading memory. Today things are different. Of course angina doesn't mean that another heart attack is imminent; nor does it mean that I can't control it with nitroglycerin tablets and continue to live a normal life. At least that's what all the books and articles tell me. They've all been written by doctors who know. Or do they? Quite suddenly it dawns on me that nowhere have I read anything written by a layman on the subject of coronary disease, detailing the personal experiences of one coronary cripple.

Is this omission due to indifference or physical impairment or lack of ghost writers? Cardiovascular diseases kill off a million people in North America each year. How come there's no word from the little people: the survivors?

Maybe we become closet cripples, fearful to admit how sick we are even to ourselves, let alone anyone else. Instead, we try to brazen it through in the best macho manner until the Big One levels us. Permanently. Who has time to write about that?

I yank the sheet from the typewriter and grind it into a tight ball, then insert a fresh page very carefully. There is something immensely satisfying in seeing a clear white page waiting for the written thought. Any thought. This day I have none.

If I still smoked this would be the ideal time to light a cigarette, contemplate the dense white acrid fumes wriggling from its lighted tip, and wait for inspiration to zap my fingers into action. But I smoke no longer. Damaged heart. Clean lungs. A martyr to medicine.

"Hi, you busy?"

Jim Armstrong pokes his head around the corner of the doorway, then comes in and puts his coffee cup on the desk edge.

"Frantic. Buried in work. Grab a pew."

He sits down with an affable smile. His job title is Inmate Counselor, which means he's a spy for the Man. Frontenac has two counselors. One for each dorm. Armstrong handles the west-dorm inmates, which makes him my counselor.

Counseling theory maintains that if irascible prisoners have a shoulder to cry on, maybe they won't erupt quite so unpredictably and destroy their premises. Or, if they are going to erupt, with any luck their counselor will have got early wind of it and be able to provide security officers with the best way to defuse the situation. It's a question of "Know Thy Enemy," and has little or nothing to do with convict welfare. But pretenses must be maintained in order to save face. There are inmate counselors within every prison in North America. This silly game of helping prisoners to reform is endemic. Both sides play the game to the hilt. One for income, the other in hopes of hastening release.

Once, Jim was an Anglican Church minister who believed in justice, the basic decency of his fellow men, and the rights of Jehovah Witnesses to make it into heaven ahead of everybody else. But after years of work in Millhaven Penitentiary and the loss of a wife to cancer, the futility of life seems to have got to him.

Jim is a big man, a gregarious, affable conversationalist with eclectic tastes, and the brightest, best-educated, and certainly the most intelligent member of the prison system I've met. But something is lacking. I feel his presence to be one of hopelessness. He seems to look on all life as a purposeless wait for death.

"We are all dying men, Tony. Remember that."

Several times he has said this to me as though it is something requiring constant reminding lest I forget myself and begin enjoying life too much for his sense of decency. He gives an avuncular smile and sits back in the chair.

"How's it going?"

This is Armstrong's standard opening and part of the reason he's ridiculed. Anything predictable is subject to ridicule within a prison. Inmates claim that he has three standard phrases which he offers as he weaves past the supplicants gathered each day outside his office door. "How's it going?", "Leave it with me," and "Have a nice day."

I decide to be obtuse. "How's what going?"

"The book."

"Nearly finished."

I know he is worried that I've put him into the story. Other staff members have told him as much, claiming to have read the draft. However, this tale has nothing to do with prison and less than nothing to do with Armstrong.

"Satisfactory ending?"

"I hope so. Satisfactory endings turn readers into customers."

He sips his coffee, trying to read the top page of typescript lying on the open file next to my Olivetti. Despite numerous visits he's never had nerve enough to ask if he could read a few pages. And I've never offered.

"Is this a social call or are you here to tell me that it's all been one huge mistake and the Parole Board have decided to cut me loose?"

Although his facial muscles tweak a smile I know he isn't laughing; nor does he think it's funny. Like every prison counselor he represents himself as the best and ultimate contact with the Parole Board, pretending that its decisions are based on his written recommendations.

This fosters a belief among prisoners that close rapport with their counselors is mandatory for positive parole consideration. But over the months I have discovered that Jim Armstrong's influence with the Parole Board is roughly the same as mine. In fact I probably have a slight edge. It's true that the Board considers a counselor's written submissions when making its decisions, but such submissions are a very small part of the whole assessment process.

"No, you haven't made parole. And if your attitude doesn't

change drastically I'm afraid you won't be getting it at all. You'll wind up doing your full time. I'm sorry, but that's how it is."

He means it. Sincerely. I want to laugh. He's talking balderdash. It's his method of countering my apparent self-sufficiency within the prison framework. I don't fit the mold, therefore I am a threat. A manipulator is an archetype created by penitentiary cognoscenti. If the system fails to manipulate you, then you become the manipulator. Simple logic. I'm a manipulator.

In fact, I was told that during the few weeks prior to my heart attack Jim told a number of other staff members that he knew I was faking and the best course to follow with my type of troublemaking was to ship me off to Millhaven and maximum security. Since January he's been trying to be friendlier.

"My dad had a heart attack," he says, looking out past my shoulder to the parking lot. "We lived out West. He was into grain heavily. Long hours, seven-day weeks trying to make his millions. When his heart attack came I thought he was going to die. I was only a kid. My dad was in his early forties, the prime of life. Looking back on it now, I think that heart attack saved him. He underwent a complete personality change afterward. Nothing was ever important enough to make him rush again. He became phlegmatic about business, politics, finances, and life in general. Quite amazing."

He shrugs and gives me a smile. "Died in his eighties a completely happy man. I guess what I'm trying to tell you is that a heart attack isn't the end of the world."

"Even a real one?"

He winces and lowers his eyes to stare thoughtfully at the typewriter. . . .

Back in November, after serving eight months of my four-year sentence, my day parole eligibility date arrived. Jim Armstrong primed me for the Parole Board hearing.

Full parole is considered at one-third of time served on a sentence, day parole at one-sixth. Both parole types are used with a carrot-and-stick approach. Remorse for crimes, religious fervor, family ties, reformation, and cunning all have a bearing on a favorable Parole Board hearing.

I have watched men go into the reviewing room with tears of remorse streaming down their faces, shoulders sloped, eyes clouded with religious mysticism as they attempt to prove their right to have another crack at society. There was one bank robber at Terminal Island who had given an act before the Board four times in as many years with the same results. Finally, no longer caring because he had less than three years left on his sentence, he stormed into the reviewing room and, after ranting and raving for fifteen minutes about what a collection of jackasses the Board members were, stormed out without giving anyone else a chance to speak. For this unusual performance he was awarded full parole when the Board called him back into the room to hear the decision. He was speechless.

From my own observations the perfect parole candidate seems to be a violent criminal who enters the system and during the first week behind bars punches out his cell mates, guards, and anyone else within swinging distance. After several weeks of subjugation in the "hole" on restricted diet and a few more vigorous punch-outs, the candidate appears to have a change of heart. This of course must be timed carefully—say, over a two- or three-year period. Fortunately most violent criminals receive sentences substantial enough to provide this degree of flexibility. By the end of his incubation period the candidate has become malleable, mellow, forgiving, even—dare I say it—yes, courteous. In short, he has reformed.

Such exemplary conduct guarantees rave reviews from counselors, chaplains, and penitentiary staff so that by the time the miscreant arrives before the Board with downcast eyes and soft-timbred tones he's practically a shoo-in. Proof positive of the benefits of a prison environment on the rehabilitation of society's misfits.

Unlike the total freedom of full parole, day parole requires candidates to live in halfway houses for months or years while they adjust to society and await their full parole date.

Armstrong insisted that I go into the Board on my knees,

begging for a chance at redemption, confessing my past crimes as mental aberrations, and swearing to change my personality and lifestyle.

"But I haven't done anything that requires an apology. In fact I'm not at all certain that someone doesn't owe me an apology."

"You were convicted," he thundered.

"So was everyone else in here, but that doesn't make us all guilty. Besides my lifestyle has been drastically altered already."

"Guilty, innocent, what difference does it make? I'm trying to get you released. You're not being very cooperative."

So I played the game this way and although the Board wouldn't give me day parole, I was given weekend releases to spend overnight at home with my family until full parole date in July. I thanked Armstrong. Would I have got it without him? Perhaps, perhaps not. Certainly his recommendations will be vastly different in July when I apply for full parole. But July is four months away and there are other more pressing things to be considered at the moment.

Surreptiously, I lift a nitro pill from the bottle in my pocket and, feigning a cough, pop it under my tongue. His presence has given me angina. Or is it because I cannot find words to type? Some stress has set the pain off again. Maddening to realize how tightly strung is this mechanism that triggers my pain. I wish Armstrong would go, leave me in peace. The pill gives a slight burning sensation as it is absorbed sublingually. In moments I can feel it working. My face and chest feel flushed. Slowly the pain recedes. I study the Olivetti, waiting. Armstrong gets to his feet and drains his coffee.

"Well, I've got work to do, so I'll leave you to it." By the door he pauses. An afterthought: "Have a nice day."

Kingston, Canada

21 May 1980

When the wires have been placed and checked for contact, I am asked to climb on a stationary bicycle and start pedaling. The doctors will measure my tolerance to exercise. This exercise room is in the old part of Hotel Dieu Hospital. High ceilings, flecking paint, plywood veneer furnishings, give it a circa Thirties dating.

A young intern is watching my graph tracings intently as I begin to pedal. Slowly at first, gradually building the stationary speed to 20 mph, where I am supposed to hold it for as long as I'm able. Within a minute I feel the first stirrings of angina. I keep pedaling. Can I make it through two minutes?

In one corner of the room is a treadmill that serves the same function as the bicycle. The young intern says that he prefers to use the treadmill but it is unserviceable at the moment.

"Has been for months. No one knows how to fix it," he explains.

I find this inconceivable. The machine looks so simple: an electric motor hooked to a reduction gear, connected to two rollers over which a wide rubber belt has been inserted. It is simple to me, while what the doctor is studying looks infinitely more complex. Each to his own.

The bicycle strikes me as far more practical anyway. A simple commercial exercise machine with few moving parts. People power instead of electrical power.

The angina gets worse. At two minutes I stop as the pain hits a crescendo. A nurse regards me anxiously.

"Uh, you okay?"

She's a redhead with freckle-splattered features and deep blue eyes. Her hand brushing my forehead is cool and soothing. I'm sweating from pain and my face is gray. A quick nod that I'm all right and she helps me off the machine and over to the bed to lie down. The intern looks quickly from me to the tracings and back again several times.

My breath is shallow and carefully controlled. I don't want to do anything excessive and hold the angina from its departure. After a couple of minutes it starts to fade. Color returns to my face. I feel better. The nurse smiles. Her left incisor is turned slightly inward. She should see an orthodontist. It's a shame to spoil such a lovely smile. Or maybe that tiny imperfection is what gives it such beauty.

"Starting to feel a bit better?" the intern asks.

He knows I am. His face has relaxed. He switches off the machine and strips away the spool of graph paper that has spilled over the floor. Do they ever lose a patient on the exercise machines, I wonder? Some poor cardiac cripple trying to test or prove his mettle against the machine, only to be leveled suddenly by a clot or a muscle spasm that chokes off the blood supply to a critical artery? I'd like to inquire but it seems as though it might be considered bad form. After all, what professional wants to discuss his failures with a layman?

I am asked to describe the pain. Where it started, how it felt, where it spread, how it departed? He writes none of it down, so I suspect that it's merely information to satisfy his own curiosity or stack away in a memory bank for later comparison to future patients.

"What happens next?" I ask.

He tilts his head. "I'll turn in my report to Dr. Burggraf and let him decide on the next step."

"How did I do?"

"Not very well, I'm afraid."

A wheelchair takes me back to my room in the new section where the surroundings feel more salubrious to survival. Two days pass.

Cardiac angiography is performed in the basement of Kingston General Hospital. Accordingly, I have to be transferred in an ambulance from Hotel Dieu for this invasive coronary procedure. It's all new to me and rather exciting, another step in finding out what is wrong, and if it can be fixed. There are mysteries to be uncovered, decisions to be made.

My feelings are similar to those when I was much, much younger and landing for the first time in some foreign country, anxious to explore its terrain and customs. Slight fear of the unknown and delicious anticipation of the new and novel. A few weeks earlier, Dr. Gary Burggraf introduced me to the idea.

"Do you know what an angiogram is?"

"No."

"I'm going to recommend that you have one when we can fit you in."

"Ah."

"There are risks, but they're minimal."

"How minimal?"

"One out of a thousand dies."

Beautiful odds. How could I argue? Burggraf has replaced the Mighty Koval as my emotional clutching post. He's a quiet, unassuming man with studious schoolmaster spectacles, thinning hair, and pale features. His voice is soothing, softer than any doctor's should be. It is impossible to believe that he could ever lose his temper and raise his voice. He explains the science of angiology in simple terms. It is a study of the lymph and blood vessels within the body.

By-pass operations begin with an angiogram. A reflective dye is injected into the bloodstream at the coronary arteries, its course followed with an X-ray scanner while being photographed. Later, doctors study the results and decide collectively on a course of action.

The principle of locating defective areas along the blood vessels had been used for many years in conjunction with the development of X-rays. However, the use of angiography for locating heart defects happened by accident in 1958 at the Cleveland Clinic. Dr. F. Mason Sones, Jr., and his colleagues were injecting an normal X-ray opaque dye into a catheter that Dr. Sones had inserted into a patient. The catheter, a long, slim, flexible tube, had been slid into the brachial artery of the right arm in front of the elbow and slipped carefully up into the subclavian artery under the collarbone. His intention had been to enter the heart through the arch of the aorta, then as usual go through the aortic valve into the left ventricle. But the catheter slipped into the right coronary artery instead of the left ventricle. Horrified by his mistake, he watched the monitor screen in fascination. Until that moment it had been thought that any foreign substance inserted into coronary arteries would cause heart instability, damage, or blockage. But his patient remained unaffected by the mistake. Medical history had been made.

Dr. Sones went on to develop a catheter that would be easier to handle in finding the coronary orifice. He discovered that the amount of injectate could be reduced, resulting eventually in his ability to reach into blood vessels as small as 100 microns, about the size of a ballpoint pen tip. Sones's catheter brought in the new era of revascularization surgery. His discoveries made possible an accurate diagnosis of coronary artery disease and, perhaps most important of all, defined the needs of individual patients.

It had taken Ted DeJager nearly a month to make the arrangements for me to see Dr. Burggraf. During that time my angina pains kept on growing, like some disgusting fungus inside my chest. I continued with the daily walks but somehow all enthusiasm for their medicinal value had vanished. A new concern appeared.

The Inderal tablets I'd been taking so faithfully began to react, slowing my heart rate to an incredible forty beats a minute. This was quite insufficient to provide needed oxygenated blood circulation during exercise. I started having blackouts. They happened during my circular walks about the camp's perimeter. The first collapse I attributed to spring flu, which had been running through the prison population. I had taken it home and given it to Helen and the children one weekend. But when I stumbled unconscious onto the pathway a second and third time less than a week later, it was apparent that something was drastically wrong. Naturally the first thing that came to mind was another heart attack or a series of small attacks.

People who have gone through the coronary experience have told me that until the age of forty-five every physical ailment is regarded as anything but a heart problem. After forty-five and a first heart attack, every twitch or physical discomfort is self-diagnosed as a coronary problem. At the time I thought the idea exaggeraged. Now I discover that it isn't.

On the first visit to Dr. Burggraf the Inderal dosages were reduced and my mind set at ease.

"Different people experience different results. There has never been a medicine made with a uniform dosage to suit everyone. Forty milligrams seems to be your maximum tolerance. You might bear that in mind for the future."

But with the Inderal reduced, the angina pains became more acute in the weeks that followed. Instead of four or five nitro tablets a day, I began popping them like peppermints in an attempt to stave off the pain. By mid-May any physical exertion produced angina symptoms. I started to panic, trapped in a carcass that appeared now to be nearing extinction. There could be no doubt that within the next few weeks or months I would become a coronary cripple, incapable of any physical effort, settled into a wheelchair waiting for my ultimate heart attack to finish the matter once and for all.

It was on the next visit that Dr. Burggraf suggested angiography to see just how badly the coronary arteries were squeezing the life blood from my wounded heart.

Kingston General Hospital is enormous. It sprawls and rises over two city blocks, overlooking lake, city, park, adjacent hospital windows, and tiny enclosed courtyards. There are vital ties to the medical research facilities and funding from Queen's University. This incestuous relationship provides an incentive for attracting the best and brilliant of the medical profession to both the hospital and the university. Yes, I'm lucky to be here.

The ambulance men roll me through underground passages, around right-angle turns, through swinging double doors until outside a wide door placarded with the word ANGIOG-

RAPHY, we pause. A nurse comes out to sign a delivery slip and I am rolled inside and lifted onto a tilting operating table.

There are two doctors, a man and woman. They claim to have done hundreds of angiograms, so I am not to worry. Until this moment I haven't; however, now there's a twinge of concern. They look so very young—late twenties, no more. A few years out of high school. Or are they young because I am getting old?

A nurse straps me onto the table, cinching the buckles tightly to keep me from rolling off when the unit is tilted. Another nurse stabs my forearm with a long needle atop what looks like a ten-gallon syringe filled with yellowish liquid. She squeezes it slowly into the wound—all of it. There's no pain nor discomfort, but the sight and thought of what's happening are repugnant.

The first nurse sets my arm on a wing table extended alongside and begins daubing the exposed flesh with an orange antiseptic solution, working carefully to insure that every spot is covered. As she works my arm goes numb. Then dead.

It's not an arm any more, but an object draped with green sheets lying next to me on the table. An orange-colored slab of convex matter. A curiosity. Nothing more.

The doctor taps the arm.

"Feel anything?"

"Nothing."

"Good," he says, "that's the way it's supposed to feel." He sits down and picks a wicked-looking scalpel from the instrument tray.

"You can watch this if it doesn't bother you. The main thing to remember is: don't move."

A nurse holds the arm and he makes a deep incision. Surface blood wells out. The other doctor wipes it away. He slices deeper, sure, deft strokes, probing for the brachial artery.

"Other hospitals use the femoral artery at the groin for catheter insertion, but I prefer to go in through the arm," he explains. "It's a shorter distance into the heart. Using the femoral artery, there's always a chance of bumping into something nasty along the way."

He doesn't explain what he means by something nasty, and I'm afraid to ask.

"Ah, got it!"

He lifts the artery into view with a curved crochet hook. I can feel its pull and tug stretching from my wrist. Odd sensation. The artery pulsates, resembling a reddish-tinged length of poor-quality macaroni. A tiny slit to open it and blood spurts high, spattering the doctor's glasses. Such incredible pressure! Quickly the other doctor presses the catheter tip into the opening, stemming the flow. She feeds it slowly through the artery. A foot of plastic flex tube vanishes into my arm. Then another. I can feel it crooking around my shoulder and under the collarbone. Another peculiar sensation. No pain, just a feeling of something moving inside.

On the monitor my arteries and heart appear in faint outline, the catheter moving across the screen in bright contrast. At the aorta the doctor pauses to adjust the X-ray scanner. Focus improves. Both doctors examine the monitor. They wear lead aprons to shield their vitals from radiation. I'm remarkedly naked under a sheet.

"When the catheter is in position we're going to inject a dye through the coronary arteries and into your heart. You ll feel a sudden flush for a few seconds. Don't worry about it. It may spread down your left side as well. Perfectly normal. Should I tell you to cough, do so at once—long and hard coughs and keep coughing until I tell you to stop. Understood?"

"Understood."

The catheter tip wiggles, dancing around the arterial entrances. Every heartbeat knocks the flexible tip about unmercifully with jolts of blood pressure. The doctor tries to enter the artery he wants, twisting and turning the slender catheter. I watch the screen, fascinated. I want to help. It's a problem of manual dexterity and requires a hobbyist's talented fingers. Three, four, six times the attempt is made, but the blood flow keeps buffeting the tip away. Finally it slips neatly into the left main coronary artery and stops.

"I'm putting in the dye now."

It comes with a sudden surge of fire and vanishes abruptly. That's all? A camera, operated by a foot pedal under the table, begins photographing the dye's progress. They tilt the table to photograph from different angles. The camera whirrs. More dye is injected. This time the burning sensation is much less. More tilts and angles. More dye. On the monitor my arteries light up like busy freeways at night. If there are any blockages or narrowings, I can't see them. Maybe this has all been a mistake and I've wasted everyone's time for nothing. How embarrassing.

Then it is over. The catheter is withdrawn, the artery stitched closed. Neither doctor will tell me the results. Time is needed to study the film clips. I press them for generalities. They turn evasive, so it must be serious. Why do doctors have this annoying habit of refusing to discuss their findings with patients except with the greatest reluctance? They explain that since I am Dr. Burggraf's patient it is incumbent upon him to explain their findings. How so? What is this medical protocol that turns physicians into bureaucratic sycophants so that patients are the last ones to know about their illnesses?

An ambulance takes me back to the Hotel Dieu and my room on the fourth floor. Mr. Sung has gone, released to his family many weeks before. Different room. Different roomie. A dark, morose man who mumbles invective over a wife who "run off with a goddamn plumber" while he was in the army. He looks much too old for the army. After hearing his story the first time I inquire when this disaster took place?

"Nineteen forty-two—late summer—the bitch was in heat."

He never remarried. Thirty-eight years with this chip on his shoulder. Talk about holding a grudge. He regards our nurses suspiciously as though each shared the blame for his marital misfortune.

"Live on the farm with my brothers now. Better to live with men than women. None of that bitching about messes and such-like!"

Both brothers are bachelors, it turns out. Maybe the

experience of their older brother scared them off the marriage market. Now the family will die out. No sons and daughters left to leave their farm, furniture, and trunks filled with memories to enjoy. Sad.

In the morning Dr. Burggraf visits to say that he's decided to keep me in hospital for a few days until a decision is made by the group.

"What group?"

"The surgeons and cardiologists who study the film footage at regular weekly meetings. Any decision to operate is made collectively."

"You've seen the film?"

"Yes, but I'm not a surgeon. Sometimes it's impractical to operate. Other times the problem isn't as serious as we thought and a change in medication can correct the trouble."

His tone is soothing but the words are bullshit. I have lived too long not to be able to recognize the vital signs of deceit: tilted head, querulous shifting eyes, and compromising smile. How I hate doctors when they do this.

But of course there is an argument which maintains that if laymen knew the true condition of their medical plight they would expire forthwith from fright. I disagree with this hypothesis, as do most of the seriously ill with whom I've spoken here in hospital. If I am unsalvageable I want to know. Conversely, if my ailments are of a minor nature, then I deserve to be told so that I can stop worrying. It is not the knowledge of our impending doom that is worrisome so much as it is the lack of knowledge.

I have come to believe that all humans have the ability to meet and accept their changing circumstances with an adaptability that nature in its wisdom has provided. How else can the existing evidence be explained? People who must journey through life cruelly deformed, blinded, deafened, or mutilated still find some inner strength to rise above their crisis, and in so doing achieve peace of mind. It is knowledge that produces this peace of mind, an embracing of reality when hope has gone.

I accept that I will never fly again and feel that solitary

tumbling freedom of the sky. I accept that my body is crippled, and my lifespan undoubtedly altered from the actuarial or biblical allotment. I accept the fact that I am physically diminished and no longer able to compete with other men my age. But I cannot accept being left in ignorance of my condition when such knowledge is available to others.

Common sense tells me that something is very wrong with my heart's function, otherwise I would have been released after the angiogram. Would I be any wiser knowing all the minute details upon which a decision will be based to operate or not? Maybe, maybe not. Certainly I'd be a lot happier knowing. But Burggraf is the doctor and the option to tell me all or nothing remains with him.

"I may have some news for you tomorrow," he says vaguely as he leaves the room.

I hope so. Anything would be better than this suspended animation. It reminds me of awaiting examination results at the end of a school year: impossible to enjoy the summer holidays in a vacuum of ignorance.

I pass the day sauntering the corridors, reading brief excerpts from stale magazines in various waiting rooms, and talking with patients and nurses. Everybody has a story to tell or complaint to register. Only a willing ear is needed to join the action.

In one sunny alcove at the end of a hall an enormous television set holds some small-fry visitors enraptured. Their parents sit flicking through paperbacks and magazines with aimless interest. A soap opera blares, filling the room—an improbable story of human greed, lust, love, insanity, and murder. The kids hang on every word. How much of it do they understand? For a while I watch, fascinated. The players can't act. The writers can't produce believable prose. The multiplicity of plots and coincidental situations are a joke. There is more human drama and comedy on this hospital corridor than any soap opera could hope to provide. One need only look.

An old woman comes from one of the rooms halfway down the hall. She is slim and silvered with carefully managed hair and dress. Outside the door she seems to shrink, her face and figure reflecting resignation to the inevitability of what she has just seen. For a minute she stands leaning with her back against the wall, her eyes intent on a spot in the middle of the corridor floor. Another woman comes from the room. Much younger. She puts an arm around the old lady. Very slowly they come toward the waiting room. Neither speaks. They sit on one of the sofas and stare blankly at the television. A single word comes to mind. Sorrow. On the screen a young model blathers about lathers for yet another unique shampoo. The old woman searches for the other's hand, their fingers meet and lock. She sighs, a long shudder of emotion that cools the sunny room. And then very quietly mother and daughter begin to weep.

After supper Helen comes to visit with the girls in tow. The girls play cards, backgammon, or sit and color. They are a year apart in age nearly to the day and entering that gangly, coltish stage before the bumps and curves of puberty and womanhood. Two completely different personalities that I helped create. Watching them now, I feel certain that they are possibly the most important thing I've managed to accomplish.

"What did the doctor say?" Helen asks.

"In a word: patience. He may have some information in the morning. How's the job?"

I don't want to talk about me. Her day will have been much more interesting. Helen has become a "balloon lady" at the local McDonald's outlet. It's a parttime job arranging children's birthday parties for hungry hordes whose parents have opted for catered cake and balloons under the golden arches, thus avoiding disasters at home. For apartment dwellers the idea must have been a Godsend. For her it is a fun thing, keeping her mind off my problems, her own fears, and offering a chance to do something productive, albeit at minimum wage. In our present financial plight every bit helps to ease the burden. Like most prisoners' wives, she is drawing Mother's Allowance. Welfare, for Christ sake! I never thought I'd live to see the day my family would be forced to survive on handouts and food that I manage to purloin from a prison kitchen.

She tells me about her day. I play a game of cards with the girls. My roomie glowers suspiciously at the three females, then at me for responsibility for their presence. But the girls are polite and full of fun and soon he is smiling and offering them bits of candy. Helen nods at him pleasantly and he blushes.

Later, when visiting hours are past and the corridor activity returns to sounds of soft-shoed nurses and hospital attendants, Dr. Rice drops by to see me. He's a Burggraf understudy now. I haven't seen him since our talk after my heart attack.

"You've spoken to Dr. Burggraf?"

"This morning."

"Did he explain the problem?"

"More or less." I decide to fake it on the reasonable assumption that he'll keep talking if I ask the proper questions. "I'm afraid I didn't grasp it completely. He was quite busy. Another patient ... Do you have time to give me the full details?"

He pulls up the comfortable chair and sets his clipboard on the side table.

"You have three coronary arteries causing trouble. One is completely shut—the one that caused your heart attack. Another is seventy percent closed—which is probably the reason for your present angina. The third is about sixty percent closed. The rest appear normal."

"Normal?" He is remarkably well informed.

"As normal as anyone else your age. The main thing is, we've identified the problem areas. You're lucky, really you are. Some patients suffer from uniform arterial stenosis—sorry, I mean a narrowing of entire passages. When that happens, there's not much we can do except suggest medication and strict diet. But in your case the plaque buildups are at specific points along the coronary arteries. An ideal situation for by-pass surgery. I can tell you that Doctor Burggraf was pleased with your angiogram results. You're a typical middle-aged by-pass candidate: right age, good physical condition, no foreseeable complications, which means an excellent prognosis for recovery. It's really too bad the problem couldn't have been diagnosed earlier we might have been able to correct the blood deficiency before you had that infarct—heart attack."

Yes, isn't it. I enjoy hearing about the prescience of hindsight. How many doctors have laid this number on how many patients over the years, I wonder?

"Then it has been decided?"

"Not quite. Doctor Salerno has to confirm the decision. He's the surgeon. Should be around to see you in a couple of days. Offhand I'd say you'll be getting some new coronary arteries. How does the idea appeal to you?"

I feel much better. He leaves to continue his rounds. The excitement of knowing that something is going to be done starts my heart pounding and stirs the angina. Quickly I reach for a nitro pill and settle the beast back in its lair.

For a while I read. My roomie snores loudly beyond the curtain shield, each breath a graveled bubble bursting obscenely upon the silence. Eventually a nurse arrives to give us the midnight pills. The snores are strangled with a sip of water.

I get a pill to ease the pain in my arm. From elbow to wrist it throbs where the artery was pulled from the surrounding flesh. Surface skin has turned an angry purple. The pill works quickly. My eyes become leaden. I switch off the lamp and drift on the night airs. Snores start up again on the other side of the bed curtain. Softly at first, gradually building in crescendo. But I am too far away to care.

A few days later, shortly after evening visiting hours end, Dr. Tomas Salerno breezes into the room accompanied by a tall, angular nurse with a very businesslike clipboard under her arm. He comes bedside and gives my hand a formal but vigorous shake, the way guest conductors greet first violinists at center stage just before the concert gets under way. He mutters something I miss.

I press his hand gingerly, vaguely conscious of the fact that it will be this hand which will be operating on me. A hand of life or death, depending on how successful he is.

He plops into a chair and leans forward aggressively. His

nurse sits apart, clipboard balanced primly on her lap, pencil poised. Salerno is a short, medium-set man with quick, clever eyes, restless hands, and smooth, baby-skinned features. On his upper lip he sports the biggest walrus handlebar mustache I've ever seen. Without effort he manages to create the impression that he's attached to some inner time fuse that is about to explode.

"You need an operation—did anyone explain what's involved?"

"Not exactly, doctor."

His eyes bore into me. "Do you have any questions?"

"How many of these have you done?"

Quick smile. "Hundreds."

"Is my case unusual?"

"Not in the least. Run-of-the-mill. No guarantees of course. Fifteen or twenty percent of the patients still have angina when it's all over. It may be for nothing." He speaks in staccato.

"What about the other eighty to eighty-five percent?"

"Complete cure."

"How long will I take to recuperate?"

"Depends on you. Sixty days to six months. I must caution you: there's a chance you'll die."

"What sort of a chance?" I'd like specifics.

"One percent."

"You're joking. You're that sure of yourself?"

"I'm sure about your odds. But you may be one of the unlucky ones. Now and again I lose a patient. Can't predict what will happen in every operation. I do my best. I'm good. One of the best in this business. What do you say?"

"I say when do you operate?"

He gives a short nod, springing to his feet like an acrobat.

"Good! I like a man who can make up his mind. I'll fit you into the operating schedule in two or three weeks. There's no emergency in your situation. Don't worry. Relax. Leave everything to me."

And out the door he goes like a destroyer's bow wave, the

angular nurse following his wake. For a moment I lie back in bed collecting my thoughts. Now that the decision has been made to operate, I feel numb from the relief of knowing. Now there is hope the angina can be corrected. Now I have something to look forward to with hopeful anticipation. I phone Helen with the news. We talk. Will they hold me here or return me to my private office at Frontenac? Will my recovery take sixty days or six months? Will I survive the ordeal? You bet I will.

A week slips past. There are too many coronary emergencies to ease me into Salerno's busy schedule. But on the first day of June I am given a date: June 16. The next morning I return to Frontenac where both good and bad news await.

The good news is a letter from Nancy Colbert, a literary agent I have never met, who tells me that Swan Song has been accepted for publication by a major international publisher, providing I agree to a number of revisions. The publisher wants the story changed from nonfiction to fiction. Apparently as a true story it was too unbelievable. The cash advance is like manna from heaven.

I had written a blind letter to Nancy Colbert from Joyceville, asking her help in selling the material I was churning out. Possibly this bizarre approach persuaded her, or maybe she felt sorry for me. In any case, she went to work. I'm very grateful.

The bad news is that Jim Armstrong has been playing games with my Parole Board hearing, scheduled for later in the month. He feels that I have outsmarted him, the prison system, and justice by cleverly maneuvering everyone and everything to suit my purpose. His written recommendation for parole is carefully guarded in tone but the inference is clear. In a face-to-face meeting he will not support me because he thinks I've cheated the system of their pound of flesh.

Eric Schwendau is going before the board too. He made it into Frontenac two months after me and managed to obtain the same latitude for monthly leaves of absence as I did. Although Eric is no more guilt-ridden or remorseful than I am, his outside circumstances are more familiar to Armstrong, and hence more acceptable. Eric's second wife is divorcing him and taking their new baby daughter to the East Coast to live. His business friends and associates have deserted him. When he makes parole he will be returning to Toronto and starting again at the very bottom of the corporate and business ladder. In every way he has been ruined.

This type of personal decimation is exactly what is expected to happen when a man is sent to prison. Loving families, untroubled children, faithful wives, and self-employed writers with heart problems and a private office are not so much oddities as outrages to the preconceptions of men on the "helping" side of the prison system.

But I have become indifferent to the entire matter and no longer am prepared to play head games or worry about the outcome. Besides, I'm convinced that we will be released on our July 31 parole date. The interests of "justice" have been served. Neither Eric nor I pose any threat to society as a whole or the judiciary in particular. A carefully orchestrated riptide of events has deposited both our shells high up on the beach. To get back into the water now is impossible. With luck, Eric will find a lady to retrieve his shell, adding it to her collection of pretty things and memories, while I try and work mine dexterously into prosaic fantasy, hoping to titillate the reading public. We will survive.

Kingston, Canada

30 June 1980

After lunch an ambulance takes us from the Hotel
Dieu to Kingston General Hospital. A tall, elegant man in a
hospital kimono rides with me. He's in his seventies. One of Dr.
Salerno's patients. He needs another valve repair to his heart.

"Another?"

"I had one done a few years ago. Starting to act up on me
again. Pesky things, heart valves."

The surgical approach for valve repair is the same as a by-
pass. At seventy will his constitution carry him through such a
massive operation? He appears unconcerned. Perhaps it's a case
of do or die and he has accepted the situation philosophically.

It's hot inside the ambulance. Hot as hell outside too.
Cobalt skies, spitball clouds laced with vapor trails from crossing
airways. I drink in the sights: birds ravaging insects, wavy heat
rising in mysterious mirage from scorched black asphalt, and
young beautiful girls dressed in colored cotton prints that turn
almost transparent, etching their undergarments when the
sun's angle catches their dresses just so.

Our driver and attendant talk of baseball and summer
cottages and the weekend good life. Neither is married and,
judging from the way they ogle the passing cotton prints, intend
to remain that way.

At the hospital we climb down onto new transport. In our
case, ambulatory patients mean those who can walk on and off
the ambulance between wheelchairs. The old man is wheeled off
in one direction, I in another to the tenth floor of one of the
adjoining annexes. I get a double room with a cluttered view of
windows and rooftops. The walls and floors are institutional
green and cream without warmth or comfort. The few other
rooms along the short corridor are filled with dying cancer
patients, each drifting mercifully on a drugged comatose

194

blanket, awaiting life's final release. Short cries of anguish puncture the afternoon silence, subsiding into incoherent mumbles when a nurse arrives to inject yet another morphine needle. Depressed, I sit on the bed and try thinking happy thoughts. It's difficult.

My June 16 operation date had been cancelled in the nick of time. Two days before I was due at hospital Dr. Salerno's nurse phoned to inquire if I had been off all drugs for two weeks? No, I hadn't. Good God, didn't I realize that the Anturan I'd been taking is an anticoagulant to prevent blood clotting? To undergo major surgery with that in my system would mean certain death. There was a two-week postponement to wait for the effects of my various pills to wear off. July 2 would be the new operating date.

The following weekend I drove with Helen to a local tennis club where McDonald's were catering a party. Suddenly the lights began to fade. Pain wrenched my chest. Another heart attack? A fast trip over to Hotel Dieu and cardiac emergency for tests, and I was back in the fishbowl on the fourth floor awaiting results of a blood-enzyme count. If the damage was too severe, there would be no by-pass operation until full recovery. Maybe never.

For two anxious days I lay waiting, trying to think positive thoughts. Finally Dr. Burggraf announced the enzyme count to be 187. Was it really possible to be that accurate? I'd had a small heart attack but nothing serious enough to postpone surgery, thank heavens. In all probability it happened through a combination of emotional stress in anticipation of the coming event and the suspension of medication.

To avoid further complications the decision was made for me to remain in hospital until the operation. I agreed, although it meant missing an appeal to the Parole Board when they sat in session at Frontenac later in the week. More frustrations to agitate my dozing angina.

At noon the next day while Helen was visiting, Armstrong dropped by with some papers for me to sign. Parole papers designed to avoid paying overtime wages for a team of guards while I was in Kingston General Hospital. KGH regulations were specific: no prisoner could be admitted without a twenty-four-hour escort. Parolees were exempt, therefore I was being awarded temporary parole.

"But don't think it means anything," Armstrong cautioned. "Frankly I can't see the Board giving you parole. I'm sorry, but that's the way it is."

He wasn't sorry, and as things turned out later in the day, that wasn't the way it was at all, but he managed to reduce Helen to tears by the time he left. I could have strangled him quite cheerfully.

A phone call from my parole officer, Randy Grooms, shortly before supper brought me back to a happier frame of mind. He confirmed that the Board had decided already on my case and given a full parole commencing July 31. Arrangements to return home instead of Frontenac for recuperation after the operation had been approved. The long years of trials and imprisonment were ended. A great load lifted from my shoulders and I began at once to make plans to leave Kingston. By week's end I was relaxed, happy, and looking forward to my appointment with Dr. Salerno and his team of miracle workers.

Now, sitting alone in a depressing room at KGH listening to the anguished cries of cancer patients, I have second thoughts about that earlier enthusiasm for Salerno's proposed slicing and stitching. A slight slip of the scalpel and I'll never awake from the anesthetic. It's still not too late to cancel this nonsense. Pack my few things, take the elevator to the main floor, out the door and into the real live world.

If I do, what are my chances? A short life spent fighting a losing battle with angina and a burden to everyone? Or perhaps one of those neat electrically operated wheelchairs to spare myself all physical exertion until finally my muscles atrophy? Would I not be better dead than living in progressive physical deterioration?

The floor nurse ushers another man into the room and introduces me. He's on the pudgy side with an open, guileless face and a magnificent head of stark white hair.

"Mr. Neary is another one of Dr. Salerno's patients. He's having a by-pass operation on Wednesday, too, so you'll have lots to talk about, won't you?"

She leaves to tend the dying. Neary sits down on the closest chair and fumbles for a nitro pill. His features take on a gray pallor. Pain. He squeezes his eyes closed, waiting. He's about my age, maybe a year or two older.

"Ah, that's better." His eyes open after a couple of minutes. "Bastard, isn't it?"

I agree that it is indeed a bastard. We begin to talk. He's in real estate, has a wife and several older children. His angina has been building for several years and although he hasn't had a heart attack yet, his angiogram showed that it would only be a matter of time. He's scared. For some reason this adds to my feelings of confidence that I have made the right decision. Salerno gave him a 93 percent survival factor, as against my 99 percent—maybe because he is a bit overweight and two or three years older. There is nothing that improves one's outlook and sense of well-being more than to talk with some other poor sod who is in much worse physical and emotional shape. I regard Neary as a gift from the gods sent for my personal benefit.

Accordingly, I start by giving him all the arguments for by-pass surgery, the success ratios, the development history, Salerno's reputation as a master craftsman, and finally the frightful alternatives with which we are both familiar. While convincing him, I'm convincing myself, using his reactions as a sounding board for arguments I have been presenting myself privately for weeks.

It must have been one hell of a sales job because by the time Neary's wife and daughter arrive to visit later in the afternoon we're both ready to sign up for heart-lung transplants should the necessity arise.

His daughter is at the pretty marriageable age. His wife, an older version of the daughter, is a big, earthy woman with an encompassing compassion and soft, concerned eyes. Later Helen turns up with our girls and the two families, drawn together by mutual misfortune, share in the make-believe lightheartedness and laughter.

Peter is off on a ten-day cruise of Lake Ontario in a square-rigged ship to see the world. Helen admits to a few tears and misgivings at dockside when he sailed away, although Peter had been much too excited, or disciplined, for any emotional displays. I intend to walk along the dock and greet him when he returns.

The next day one of the cancer patients dies, an old man who fails to answer the nurse's needle call. I had seen him the day before, staring vacantly at the flaking sky over his bed. He appeared well into his eighties, a tall man with patrician features and ragged military mustache bristling from a thin, pale lip. Several times the nurse tries rousing him. The various tubes running in and out of his body are dripping urine, blood, pus, sucrose, and water. But he is quite dead.

Attendants come and clean away the evidence, scrubbing the bed, floor, and walls, so that by lunchtime the room is ready to receive its next occupant. Neither Neary nor I feel very hungry.

"Just as well," the nurse says professionally. "Solid foods have to leave your body as solid waste. It's going to be several days after your operation before you'll be able to have a bowel movement."

For supper we drink fruit juice. Wives and children come to visit. The girls climb on my bed while Helen takes flash photos for mementos—or memories, depending how things work out in the morning. I sign another Will, which seems a bit silly since what little I owned was transferred to Helen years before.

The evening is interspersed with a variety of visitors come to deliver instructions, encouragement, and advice. Dr. Salerno is first, coming into the room at a trot, followed by a lovely-looking nurse whom he introduces as his assistant. Carol Harkness sets out the ground rules for morning: "You'll go down first, Mr. Foster. Mr. Neary, we'll take you next at about eleven-thirty. Both of you try to get a good night's sleep."

There's a brief demonstration on the proper method for coughing after the operation. A pillow is clutched and held against the chest, then squeezed in synchronization with the cough in order to keep the wired breastbone from flexing during its healing.

When visiting hours are nearly over, a gorgeous strawberry-blond nurse appears in the doorway like a hesitant gazelle. Her face and figure are designed to cause cardiac fibrillation.

"I'm Darby Honeyman," she tells the room. "I'm a physiotherapist." She looks at us uncertainly.

With a name and figure like hers, why bother announcing a profession? Someone should send her around the wards performing deep-breathing exercises to ginger up the terminally ill.

But she is all business. What she has to tell us is of critical importance, so we must pay strict attention. I'm all ears—and eyes.

"Well now, when you come out of the anesthetic you're going to have a breathing tube in your mouth and down your throat so's you don't swallow your tongue. You won't be able to speak, and you're going to be very weak. Well now, we've developed a series of four finger signals for you to communicate. One finger raised means that you are in pain. Two fingers raised indicates that you are thirsty. Three means that you want to cough, and four fingers tells the nurse that you want your back adjusted. Well now, are there any questions?"

I have a dozen to ask, but not in front of the children. She conducts a practice session, questioning us closely to make certain that our finger lessons are digital-perfect. After my constant errors become obviously nothing but a ploy to keep her charms beaming in my direction, she departs in a rhapsody of breathless beauty to provide succor elsewhere on the premises.

The families leave. Lights are turned out. Nothing to drink after midnight. But by then both Neary and I are fast asleep. Dreamless sleep. Black shadows. No definitions. No regrets.

I'm awake shortly after dawn. Very quietly I slip down to the end of the corridor and stand at the window high above the earth, watching the birth of day. Sun, heat, water, trees, birds, sky. Life.

I remember, I remember,
the house where I was born . . .

They come for me at seven-thirty. Two jocular young men with clear, untroubled eyes and hasty hearts. Helen appears. She rides the elevator with me. Her hands are icy and trembling. No words. What is there to say? At the entrance to the operating theaters she is led away to a waiting room reserved for next-of-kin—or bereaved. While Salerno operates she will wait. For her, it will be a long wait. Mine will be over in the twinkling of an eye once the anesthetic takes hold.

On the last corridor of my journey four lines of a Kipling verse come charging into my consciousness. I learned them as a boy, not really understanding exactly what they meant. Now their meaning is perfectly clear:

> *Unless you come of the gypsy stock*
> *That steals by night and day,*
> *Lock your heart with a double lock*
> *And throw the key away.*

When I signed the hospital's release form yesterday, I handed Salerno the key to my heart. Never have I been happier to have been born a gypsy.

Without question the leader in the development of aorto-coronary artery by-pass surgery was Dr. René Favaloro, an Argentinian. In 1967 in the city of Cleveland, Dr. Favaloro used a leg vein and graft to achieve coronary by-pass. Others had tried different methods. In Canada, Arthur Vineberg had persuaded the medical world that his theory of mammary implant worked in correcting deficiencies in coronary circulation. With Vineberg's procedure a mammary artery was taken from the chest wall and stuck at random into an area of heart muscle. Some of the blood that escaped from the artery into the wall of the heart muscle did provide a small by-pass. Dr. Favaloro, on the other hand, used a length of vein to by-pass the artery block after determining its exact location through the use of new sophisticated angiography.

Coronary artery by-pass became known as "open-heart surgery" because it required the use of a heart-lung by-pass machine, although the heart itself rarely had to be opened.

Hospital mortality was extremely low and patients' relief from angina quite spectacular. Favaloro's operational methods proved so popular that by 1982 over one million successful by-pass operations had been performed in North America. For any major block in the left main coronary artery—known as the "widow-maker"—Favaloro's operation was all but mandatory.

Dr. Favaloro returned to Argentina with a medal presented to him by the American College of Cardiology. Its inscription read: *This man's fierce patriotism to his native country cost the United States one of the finest surgeons in the world.*

It is perhaps presumptuous for a layman to describe the medical procedures for by-pass surgery. Dr. Favaloro's published papers are available through any medical library. However, they are written by a surgeon for use by surgeons and require considerable translation and explanation in order to be understood by a vast majority of the reading public, myself included. Nonetheless, it is useful to understand the basics of the procedure in order to appreciate some of the postoperative effects that can result in different people for a variety of different reasons.

Once the darkness clamps down and the patient's body goes limp, the surgeons go to work quickly. Needles from elevated bottles of sodium Pentothal and glucose are slid into arm veins and taped securely; two others inserted into the wrists record the venous and arterial blood pressures. Electrocardiogram leads are attached to the patient's extremities. At two-inch intervals under the scalp electroencephalogram needles on yellow, green, and red wires are placed, the last attached to the left earlobe.

Once connected, all impulses from the heart and brain and blood vessel pressures are collected in a polygraph machine. The patient's life signs are recorded on graph paper and projected simultaneously onto a television monitor. Thus the surgeons have an instant running profile of their patient's condition at all times during the operation.

A curved plastic breathing tube is inserted into the patient's mouth over the tongue and down into the throat. A lubricated catheter is slipped through the penis into the bladder. Anesthetic causes the sphincter muscles to relax, resulting in an annoying continuous urine drip from the patient onto the operating table. With a catheter attached, the discharge dribbles into a plastic bag under the table.

A small steel plate is slipped under the patient's buttocks to ground against electrical shocks when the Bovie electric needle is used to cauterize the tiny veins and blood vessels that are sliced during the operation. Surgeons call them bleeders and they can be very annoying when a doctor is trying to perform precise delicate needlework through layers of syrupy blood.

Finally a scrub nurse swabs the patient from a small basin of Mercresin antiseptic, covering everything from neck to thighs and down the right leg to the ankle. A towel draping is placed between the legs and over a heavy wire cage at the head. The entire body is covered except for a narrow rectangle of yellow-stained chest.

Lines from the heart-lung machine are anchored to the edge of the table. The machine looks like a small apartment-sized washer with a side-loading glass door. It sits atop a panel of rotary pumps. Without the development of this machine, open-heart surgery would be impossible.

The machine is primed with a cold cocktail mixture of glucose and water that works as well as whole blood, with the added advantage that it tends to reduce any risk of secondary infection that might be caused by using whole blood. When in operation, it will lower the patient's body temperature to 28 degrees C. (82.4 F.) and at the same time cleanse the blood of carbon dioxide and inject oxygen during its frothy journey through the pumping system. Heparin is added to prevent clotting while the blood is being circulated outside the body.

When operating, the machine pulsates, rather than producing a steady pressure flow. The body's blood vessels were designed for pulsation delivery, so when early experiments with a constant flow pressure system produced tiny strokes, brain damage, and other vascular complications, the pulsation method was adopted.

One last check on the patient's pupil dilation to insure that he's completely under, a glance at the polygraph and monitor, and the surgeons are ready. Lights dim momentarily, then brighten as the operating room is switched over to emergency power.

Holding the patient's skin taut below the throat with thumb and index finger, the surgeon makes a deep incision running the length of the breastbone and exposing a thin layer of yellow fat under the surface skin. Blood wells up from the wound. Spurting bleeders are clamped and tied, the smaller ones cauterized with the Bovie needle.

Once the opening is dry the surgeon is ready to use the bone saw. Blue smoke and fine white dust whine from the blade as the sternum is split from bottom to top. Quickly, the open marrow is sealed with beeswax to protect it.

A heavy-duty stainless-steel retractor is fitted against the jutting edges of the rib cage. Slowly the retractor is cranked open until a full nine-inch opening is achieved. It seems quite incredible that something doesn't snap or rupture during this brutal performance. Fortunately the ribs are not anchored at the back, only in front, attaching to the breastbone with heavy gristle. Ribs have been designed by nature to flex with every breath. In time this wrenching intrusion by the retractor will repair itself.

With the chest open the lungs are visible, their pink mottled surface lying flat and glistening. Now that the thoracic vacuum has been broken, the patient can no longer breathe. One of the attendant surgeons squeezes a rubber bladder rythmically, forcing oxygen down the patient's tracheal tube. He must continue to operate this bladder until switch-over to the heart-lung machine is completed.

Pressing the lungs aside, the surgeon lifts the pericardial membrane encasing the heart and very carefully slits it open. Beneath, the dark muscle of the heart stirs with metronomic regularity.

Next, the large cava veins that transport unoxygenated blood to the heart are cut. A tourniquet holds the first while a small curved clamp closes off half its diameter. A purse-string suture is made, followed by an incision into the middle of the sewn vein where a plastic catheter from the heart-lung machine is inserted. The purse strings are drawn tight, holding the catheter in place. In similar fashion, a second catheter is placed in the other cava vein. A smaller tube is inserted into the femoral artery at the patient's groin for the return of oxygenated blood from the heart-lung machine.

The patient's left arm is flushed with heparin to keep the blood from clotting in the machine. One last check is made to insure that every clamp, needle, drip, and monitor reading is as it should be.

The surgeon flicks a switch and the rotary pumps begin turning on the heart-lung machine. Catheter clips are removed from the cava and femoral vessels and blood unfolds like a red bougainvillea behind the heart-lung window. A single right-angle clamp closes off the aorta above the heart. The great muscle stretches for an instant. Quivers. And stops. At this moment blood flow into the femoral artery changes from dark to brilliant red. Oxygenation and circulation of the patient's blood has been turned over to a machine. Technically the patient is dead.

A cold watery solution is used to preserve the lifeless heart at 4 degrees C. (39.2 F.) during the operation. This mixture retards the process of decomposition longer than if the organ were to remain dry throughout the period. Now time is of the essence, to quote the phrase that lawyers love to use so indiscriminately. Two hours on the machine is maximum before problems start to develop. Our higher senses of sight, balance, memory, and coordination can suffer through neurological insufficiencies too tiny to observe or diagnose exactly. Flesh and bone exposed too long to the open air begin to die a little and cannot be replaced or rejuvenated. The surgeons must work swiftly and efficiently.

While one surgical team works at the chest area, another is operating on the patient's right leg, slicing an opening from groin to ankle in order to remove a yard of vein. Legs have an abundance of veins that provide adequate circulation even when one or two are removed. This, too, is a delicate job. Vein endings must be closed off both in the leg and in the portion that is removed for use as the coronary by-pass. Each juncture and branch will be securely sealed against the blood pressure that will surge through once it becomes a new coronary artery. One leak could be fatal.

Veins and arteries are equipped with a valving system that maintains blood flow in one direction only. The vein removed from the leg must be reversed when installed as a coronary artery or its natural metering system will obstruct the blood flow.

Although the vein is not much thicker than a knitting needle, it is much more elastic than the coronary arteries and will stretch without difficulty to accommodate the new pulsating blood pressure from the heart muscle. In time the vein will suffer the same effects of plaque and narrowing as the coronary arteries, but this will take many years. By that time the body into which the vein has been placed will be approaching the end of its active life when everything begins breaking down.

The vein is cut into six-inch lengths for each graft. If the patient is short-legged and requires five by-passes instead of the usual three, veins will be taken from both legs.

A nurse slips a pair of 2X-power eyeglasses onto the senior surgeon's face and delivers the first piece of vein together with a curved needle and No. 3 silk thread. The veins are connected first to the coronary arteries a short distance ahead of the blockages or restrictions that were discovered in the angiogram. A smooth, tiny hole is scalpeled at each coronary junction for the vein to be inserted, then sewn into position. A sealant keeps it from leaking until the graft takes root in the artery during the first week after the operation.

The veins are then connected to the aorta while heat is being returned gradually to the heart. It's slow, exacting work requiring infinite patience and an incredible manual dexterity. Some surgeons can work swiftly, whipping the stitches into place faster than any seamstress. Others take longer. Speed is essential. The shorter the time spent on the heart-lung machine, the less likelihood there is that postoperative complications will develop. But speed and accuracy are the result of constant practice, which is why hospitals that specialize in coronary by-passes have fewer postoperative problems and a higher success rate than those institutions which offer patients a more general program of care.

As work on the chest progresses, the lower team stitch the patient's leg together and slip on an elastic stocking to hold the incision and prevent any pooling of blood from stray bleeders caused by muscle movements.

After the grafts are attached, the patient is ready to be taken off the heart-lung machine. Twenty cc. of Protamine are injected into the pump to counteract the anticoagulant adminis-tered earlier.

The first cava vein is reconnected and the clamp above the aorta removed. Blood fills the heart. This is the critical moment for surgeons and patient. No matter how many similar operations they perform, every cardiac surgeon admits to tension and a considerable degree of awe when he gazes down at that inert mass of muscle and waits for its first stirrings of rebirth.

It starts as a quiver. Brain signals are triggered as the organ fills with blood. Another quiver. Then a beat. Then another. Suddenly it awakens. Its steady rhythm resumes. Everybody relaxes.

Each of the grafts is checked carefully. One by one the rotary pumps for the heart-lung machine are shut down as the heart takes over. Catheters are removed from the remaining cava vein and femoral artery. The incisions are stitched closed. A nurse turns off the heart-lung machine. It's time to close up shop.

First the pericardium membrane is stitched loosely to-gether so that any fluid that might collect can drain into the chest cavity for absorption instead of pressing against the heart. The retractor is released, bringing the two halves of the breastbone together. Both sides are cleaned of beeswax before being tied securely into position with stainless-steel wire. Finally the flaps of chest skin are sewn back into place and the patient is ready for removal to the recovery room and intensive care for at least twenty-four hours while his metabolism adjusts.

Any major surgery plays havoc with the body's chemical balances. Liver, kidneys, and pancreas are affected. Sugar, potassium, salt, and fluid levels fluctuate wildly. The body needs time to recover. Some bodies can't and go into shock. Recovery depends as much on the patient's age, physical constitution, and mental outlook as it does on the administration of bedrest and medication. Some operations are completely successful, but the patient dies a few hours or days later for no apparent reason. Others confound the odds and survive. No one can tell which category they will fall into until the deed is done, the anesthetic begins wearing off, and the beat of life resumes.

Kingston, Canada

2 July 1980

Consciousness arrives in a hazy abstract pattern of overhead lights, bright windows, gleaming metallic bed frames. And pain. Pain is everywhere. My brain and eyes are locked within this pain and fighting to float above it. The effort of sight tires my eyes. I shut them for a moment. Or many minutes? Time is no longer capable of measurement, nor I of measuring time.

When I focus again, the patterns are no longer hazy but filled with sharp definitions. There are nurses moving beside the bed, adjusting things, fussing, murmuring. A great relief floods through me. I have survived! I'm alive! Oh my, the wonder of it all.

Here I am in pain, immobile in bed, bristling with needles and tubes and pissing into a bag, but goddammit I'm alive. I'll be a sonofabitch!

Confession time.

Ninety-nine to one—those were Salerno's odds. But lately I've become a pessimist. Realistically I figured my odds to be fifty-fifty. Not because I thought Salerno was a liar, but with the way my luck has been running, mine would be the operation he started with a hangover and for the first time managed to drop that whirling saw into a patient's heart—or hooked the by-passes up backward.

With great effort I move my head. They have my bed cranked up so that I'm sitting instead of lying flat. Just as well, too, because my backache would have to be experienced to be believed. The room is fitted for four beds and a small desk for the nurse. One bed is missing. In its place is a chair. Helen is sitting on it. Her eyes watch with wonder. I try to smile but the damn tube stuffed down my throat makes this impossible. How to signal her that I'm all right, that everything is going to be fine, not to worry because I'm alive? My hands are too weak to lift. Instead I wink.

Her smile of relief fills the room with sunshine. I begin to cry. No reason really. Perhaps they are tears of happiness and salvation, the knowledge that someone I love is close enough to touch and care.

For a time I drift, dozing in and out along the warped edge of reality, trying to assemble thoughts. So many thoughts that need examination. It's difficult because my mind persists in wandering away down cul-de-sacs of trivia. I must take hold and discipline myself to think only of what is important. But how to decide?

They've given me drugs for pain. I can feel these various insidious chemicals coursing through my cold bloodstream, affecting my equilibrium. At times I am spinning around and around and around high in the sky, out of control. Then it all changes abruptly and I'm falling down ... down ... down.

There's a punctuating noise. A familiar tempo of hollow sound followed by a soft hiss. An oxygen mask? Of course. How stupid of me. I'm breathing oxygen because we're flying above ten thousand feet. Violent thunderstorms bolting jagged tears of white, blinding light come crashing through the night. Rain squalls slash the windshield; ice pellets hammer the radar nose cone like buckshot on a tin roof. I'm fighting to hold the wings level but it's no use. According to all our flight panel instruments the aircraft is out of control.

I want to scream but can't. I'm suffocating. Smothering to death. I have to cough. Just a short, sharp cough to clear away the accumulated phlegm and maybe I'll survive. My eyes snap wide. Cough? From somewhere I remember someone giving me instructions if I needed to cough. There's a coughing signal, isn't there? Well of course there is!

Dear, sweet, pneumatic Darby Honeyman. Slowly ... very, very slowly my right hand rises from the sheets, three of its fingers clearly extended. A nurse materializes bedside. A sweet, dimpled matron with understanding gray eyes.

"There, there now," she soothes. "Try to relax. You're going to be all right." She presses my hand back on the sheet.

Relax? Is the woman mad? Of course I'm going to be all right if she'll just take this goddamn tube out of my throat so that I can cough and breathe and talk. Another try with the three fingers pointed accusingly at her face. Is she blind? Stupid?

Again she places my hand on the bed and this time holds it from further movement. And speaks sharply: "Really, you must control yourself or you'll pull out all your I.V.s."

This fat, beady-eyed harridan with the mustached lip has made up her mind to kill me. He survived the operation, doctor, but a nurse did him in when he reached the recovery room. Bad luck. Still, we did our best.

Helen sits where I left her on the other side of the room, but she is too far away to help. She speaks to the nurse. I miss the words because of the buzzing in my brain. I'm thirsty, too. God, I'm dry!

I try two fingers aloft, holding them high triumphantly like a pair of talismans. But the nurse only reaches across the bed to knock my left hand into inarticulate submission. Right hand. Left hand. It makes no difference. I'm doomed.

Time struggles by on creaking wooden axles.

"You awake?"

I open my eyes. Dr. Salerno examines me with a trace of amusement. One of his walrus mustaches is askew. He's dressed in operating greens and wearing a ridiculous skullcap. Behind him, and blocking my view of Helen, is the missing bed. In it at the same tilt as my own is Mr. Neary. He looks ghastly. Maybe he's dead already? If not, I wouldn't give ten cents for his chances of survival.

"I gave you three by-passes. Made a new man out of you. Don't try any cartwheels for a day or two."

I try making some appreciative gurgling noises.

"Nurse, take that tube out of his mouth. He's awake."

Dear good generous understanding compassionate Dr. Salerno. My first reaction when the tube is gone is to cough. I forget the pillow-holding instructions and crank out a nicely rounded phlegmy bark.

Disaster!

The sudden pain is indescribable. It feels as if my entire upper works have blown apart.

"Now that was foolish, Mr. Foster. You've supposed to hold a pillow over your chest if you want to cough," says the nurse tartly. "Weren't you given proper instructions by the hospital physiotherapist?"

Dr. Salerno examined the blood bag hanging from the side of my bed. The bag is fed by two large plastic tubes that have been inserted into my chest cavity under the rib cage. A steady flow drains into the bag. And there seems to be a hell of a lot of blood in that bag. Too much?

I watch Salerno's face for signs. His brow furrows. Has a by-pass ruptured or torn loose from the aorta so that I'm bleeding to death? Plasma coming in through my arms, life blood draining away into a plastic bag. Wonderful.

I whisper: "It is serious?"

Salerno looks up, startled. "Let me worry about this situation. You worry about getting better. That way we won't worry each other."

Good advice. But it doesn't help. I'm still worried.

I drowse and doze. The trickle slows to a steady drip. Night comes to the room. Helen has left. I'm tired. I sleep.

Day Two. Quite perceptibly I'm better. Stronger. My arms can move and with careful toe work against the end of the bed I'm able to stop the annoying slippage caused by the bed's angle.

A new design for hospital shirties is needed. Velcro backs that could be attached to Velcro sheets and prevent patients from bed slippage. Even the slightest movement causes a slide over the sheets which, if left unchecked, would deposit the patient in a ball at the end of the bed. I'm sure that Velcro is the answer.

I'm still unable to lift myself bodily or change positions. That requires help from the nurse. Surprisingly, it is not the chest area where my pain is centered but rather in my back. A frightful backache has resulted from the rib cage being pushed out of position. Constant adjustments are necessary to find a few minutes' relief.

Neary is having the same problem. He gives a wan smile. Remarkably, he looks a great deal better than he did yesterday. In fact I'd be willing to say now that he will live providing there are no complications.

Postoperative complications. A horrible phrase. Enough to strike fear into the stoutest heart. Doctors use it on next-of-kin to explain the reason their patient died. Massive bleeding, shock, pneumonia, secondary heart attack—take your pick. "Postoperative complications" provides a grab bag of possibilities for the obituary notices. And it sounds so creditable.

Shortly after dawn Salerno marches into the room, conferring with a pair of doctors. The man is a phenomenon. When does he sleep? The duty nurse comes to her feet and hands him a clipboard of hourly temperature and blood pressure checks. One of the doctors removes my oxygen mask and holds it against his ear.

"Aha. Thought so. No wonder your blood oxygen hasn't been responding. This isn't working. You've been breathing air from the exhaust openings all night."

While I slept they had been sending blood samples away for examination. According to the results I was suffocating to death very slowly. He appears tremendously pleased by the discovery.

"Here, see for yourself."

He thrusts the mask against my ear as if I'd been on the point of arguing the matter. How many patients has the hospital managed to suffocate over the years? The thought angers me, but what the hell. It's not his fault that the equipment didn't work. He hangs the mask on a wall knob and bends to examine the blood bag with Salerno.

"Bleeding's stopped. Time to disconnect."

My chest tubes have been taped into position. Salerno grabs the lot and pulls everything smoothly. There's no pain but I blink with surprise at the length of these tubes. At least twelve inches of hollow plastic have been resting inside me.

Next, the urine catheter is cut and removed from my bladder. Its passage stings, and for a day or two afterward urinating is very painful.

Two needles are removed from my arms. Two remain in place. I'm nearly weaned.

Breakfast arrives. Sip of juice. Two spoonfuls of cereal. I'm exhausted. Weird how weak I've become. Never in my life have I felt so weak and incapable of physical effort. Often, ending a road race or a one-hour swim, I have felt exhausted and lain gasping for breath, my heart hammering a violent staccato. But in such cases there was no weakness, only lack of air, which could be recovered quickly with rest. But this is different and a little alarming. Recovery of my senses is progressing satisfactorily, but the incredible weakness feels exactly the same now as when I awoke after the operation yesterday.

Helen visits in the afternoon after lunch. I ate nothing. Nor do I feel much like talking, thinking, or doing anything beyond concentrating on rest. It's selfish, I know. She wants to know that I'm feeling better, hear me say the words. Perhaps a joke or wry comment. Anything. But I can't.

One of the empty beds is rolled out and a few minutes later Dr. Salerno and his team escort it back into the room. On it is the old man who rode with me in the ambulance from the Hotel Dieu. They've given him a new heart valve.

I examine his condition with an experienced eye. Even asleep he looks better than Neary did. But he's losing a hell of a lot of blood. In fact it is literally pouring into the plastic bag. The doctors watch it. Five minutes pass. The flow remains the same.

"We've got a leaker," Salerno announces. "Okay, let's take him back and open him up again."

And they all return to the operating room. Poor old man. I know he can't survive a second opening. The shock will kill him. His wife leaves with the doctors, she is weeping softly. Within the hour they roll him back—alive. I'll be damned.

Evening purples the windowpanes. Helen departs. Thirty hours have passed. No complications so far. I have this feeling of fullness in my chest, as if I've been stuffed with eiderdown.

Strangely, the worst pain is still in my back. My chest hurts much less than I thought it would. How very odd. Perhaps there are few nerves at the sternum to cause pain. Comparing this with broken ribs, which I remember immobilized me completely for three days, I'd place the pain from a split sternum at least 50 percent less. Is there such a thing as a pain chart for operations so that patients can anticipate in advance the sort of pain they're likely to encounter by comparing it with a pain with which they are familiar? If there isn't, there should be.

I eat a little supper. Liquids mostly. Chewing uses too much energy. Now I need to pee. The nurse brings a metal beaker. I adjust it under the covers. No luck. My bed position has shut off the critical valve. Cautiously I wriggle around until both legs hang from the edge of the bed and I'm sitting upright. The valve opens and a torrent fills the cannister. It burns like the devil.

Well now. I must be getting stronger because I couldn't have done that this morning. Progress is measured by accomplishment. A series of tiny triumphs. The nurse is unimpressed and orders me back on the sheets.

"Hey, Neary. How do you feel?"

"Terrible," he admits.

"Me too. It's the shits, isn't it? But y'know something?"

"What?"

"We're alive."

Sometime in the middle of the night the old man's heart stops. I awake to see nurses and doctors clustered around his bed. All working frantically to restart the circuitry. They pound and press his chest.

Jesus. Sweet Jesus. I can feel his hurt from here.

Nothing. No bleep on the cardiac monitor. A doctor sticks a needle into his chest while another touches electrodes to his body. At each power jolt the old man jerks, stiffening like a monster in a horror movie. Four, five, six times he goes rigid. His heart starts beating. Slow, steady peaks and valleys shine in fluorescent triumph from the monitor. Minutes pass. The crowd bedside break up, leaving instructions for the night nurse to keep a close watch. Neither Neary nor I get so much as a sympathetic glance when they depart. At forty hours post-op, we're well out of the woods and standing on the meadow's edge. I go back to sleep.

Day Three. A big breakfast because I'm hungry. Good feeling. Good sign, the nurse says. Across the room, the old man is awake. He stares at the ceiling with unblinking eyes. His catheters are still connected, although the leakage of blood has stopped. He's a tough old sonofabitch, that one.

Midmorning Salerno nips in for a fast check on the old man. He's still wearing operating-room greens. Only once have I seen him out of them, when he came visiting at Hotel Dieu. He must live in his greens.

"You two are moving to Victory 2. I need your bed space."

Before either Neary or I can speak, he's gone. A short time later attendants arrive with wheelchairs. We're assisted off our beds. Gigantic effort. Exhausting.

Brown file envelopes are set on our laps—something to hang onto for the trip. Waves and thanks to our nurses. As I start feeling better they have become more gentle and considerate of my complaints and pains. A tiny trick of mind? They do their jobs with unbelievable dedication and compassion.

We're off. A labyrinth of busy corridors that stretch into infinity, past doors, in and out of elevators, around corners until at last we arrive at our destination. Neary peels off into one four-bed room while I am wheeled into a smaller double room farther down the corridor.

Large hospitals suffer from the disease of expansionitis. It's incurable. It begins with a well-designed hospital of efficient contemporary design flanked with wide, rolling lawns spotted by tall shade trees. Soon it isn't big enough. A piece of the lawn disappears under a six-story annex. Five years later a ten-story wing slices through a cluster of the shade trees to become the new West Annex. Through the years growth continues unabated until the lawns, trees, and surrounding streets are swallowed by a jumble of crazy shapes, internal designs, and strange names. Names like annex, east and west block, or wing are forsaken for more politically acceptable and majestical captions: "Mackenzie King Wing" or "Duke of Edinburgh Block" or "Victory."

In such cases the age of these various additions can be determined with a reasonable degree of accuracy. The "Mackenzie King Wing" is definitely pre-World War II. "Duke of Edinburgh Block" places it in the early Fifties, while "Victory" is a product of the mid-Forties. The Golden Years when everything was possible.

It would be hard to imagine a more dreadful place from which to recover from any surgery than on the second floor of "Victory." A penitentiary cell would be preferable. At least in a cell one is permitted solitude, and help, if needed, is only a whisper away from the men on either side.

My room looks as ill as its other patient, a man who is dying of some particularly insidious form of cancer. The walls have been chipped and bashed and painted a hundred times with a hundred different colors. Overhead lighting is a pale sickly yellow. A single dirty window looks out across a dreary scene of more dirty windows. Floor tiles are cracked and split, a few curling at the corners. The toilet drips incessantly with a sound from a dungeon nightmare. Furnishings are very old, providing a sort of functional indifference instead of pleasant amenity. Victory 2 is a crypt for worn-out bodies, tired decaying minds, and hopeless souls. A place for dying. No one wants to be here, nurses or patients.

The attendant helps me onto the bed. A skinny nurse watches suspiciously. She has mean little black eyes set on a small square face. The attendant gives her the brown envelope and together they leave, the nurse complaining loudly about missing her coffee break. I scrunch down in the bed feeling miserable.

But by evening Helen has me laughing so hard that my chest feels as if the tie-wires have unraveled. It's laughter of relief, slightly hysterical, an emotion seeking a reason to blossom and flower. The reason is Helen's description of my absurd and pathetically weak hand signals given as I came out of anesthetic; Darby Honeyman's guarantee to physical comfort and survival.

We roar with laughter until tears roll down our cheeks. Two nurses appear at the doorway and stand with mouths agape. Laughter on Victory 2? No one ever laughs on Victory 2. No one would dare!

Day Four. My roomie spent the night in delirium. Apparently it is the chemicals they're giving him. He's just had an operation to kill his brain's pain awareness. The cancer has spread everywhere, so they give him chemotherapy. If the cancer doesn't kill him the chemicals will if he's lucky.

A case in point: Glen Veley, Frontenac's senior cook, learned that he had lung cancer this past November. Too far advanced to operate; so the doctors prescribed a combination of horseshit and hope: chemotherapy. He believed in hope. Veley taught me the rudiments of creating pastry. A crude hard-living man but intensely loyal, even lovable once the surface facade was penetrated. We became close friends. Jailer and convict. I was astonished by his cooking talents, most of them unappreciated by the prison's staff and cons. Veley was a master chef who could create miracles in a kitchen.

Every year he took his wife to Florida for a holiday. In April, on their way home from Daytona, he had a massive arterial explosion, hemorrhaged, and suffocated in his own blood. What killed him, the cancer or the chemicals? I never read his death certificate and Jim Armstrong refused me permission to attend the funeral.

In life, Veley and Armstrong always seemed to be at each other's throats. I was always sorry to have missed the sight of Jim Armstrong on his knees in church praying for Veley's immortal soul.

Shifts change in the early dawn. A new nurse makes medication rounds. Never the same nurse. Victory 2 is considered hardship assignment for nurses. No volunteers. Administration conscripts, the lot of them.

I receive Digoxin to settle the rhythmic balance of my

heart, a tiny diuretic pill that causes me to pee gallons, and a small paper cup of liquid potassium mix to replace the potassium loss caused by the diuretic. All rather like a dog chasing its own tail to my way of thinking. Apparently it is necessary to flush away the rapid buildup of body liquids that appear after surgery. Such flushing process removes much of the body's potassium, which must be replaced immediately.

My chest still feels full of feathers but the back pains are easing at last. Thinking processes are back to normal, although emotionally I feel on the verge of tears. When I tried speaking last night to Salerno to thank him for his effort my voice cracked and I nearly broke down. Embarrassing. Maybe it's something they have given me which causes this reaction. The feeling is constant. I see that poor bugger in the next bed and know that I am going to live while he must die, even though we're the same age. I think how lucky I am to have been born late enough in the century to receive an operation that was perfected in time to save my life. Every thought brings a feeling of gratitude and awareness such as I have never felt before, and behind every thought sits a rain barrel of tears waiting to flow. Hopefully this feeling will pass sufficiently that I will not leave the hospital a blubbery wreck mumbling maudlin choke phrases. I must get a grip on myself.

After breakfast and doctor's rounds I am encouraged to try walking. So soon? Well, why not? The first trip is a cautious seven wobbly steps to the bathroom. Ten thousand miles as the crow flies. I sit down and mount a mighty effort to relieve five days of accumulated bowel pressure. Can't be done. The slightest strain, halfhearted heave, or muscular contraction cause indescribable pain across my chest.

Exhausted, I sit contemplating alternate courses of action. Everything is sitting there, just aching to leave the premises but I'm incapable of helping it along. It's really quite infuriating.

I hunch forward, changing the passage angle. Nothing. A few minutes of sitting bolt upright waiting for the force of gravity to take over likewise produces nothing tangible. I'm determined not be defeated. Patience. The waiting game. The power of positive thought. Think of pleasanter things. Butter-flies on a summer day. Sunflowers nodding in an afternoon breeze. And the sign on the door in front of my eyes: IN CASE OF EMERGENCY RING FOR THE NURSE. Just what in hell she could do about my present predicament isn't mentioned.

Minutes pass. There's a tiny perceptible movement, a stirring of anticipation. A knock at the door interrupts this concentration: "Are you all right in there."

A statement, not a question. When I need a nurse, a steady ring on the bed buzzer for fifteen or twenty minutes will produce nothing more than an aching thumb. Now when I'm trying to think positive, all of a sudden my bathroom welfare becomes the paramount issue for the entire floor. I can hear two—no, three—of them out there discussing me in anxious tones.

"Fine."

One word I give them. They're entitled to that. Then they're on their own.

"If you need help, remember to ring."

They depart. More minutes pass. Sweat beads my brow. Now I have a new pain. A tearing pain. Success! The relief of that backlog more than compensates the rip it causes. I sit in happy rapture, allowing every problem to slide away. With all the pills, injections, and medicines I'm being given why didn't someone think of a tablet for constipation?

Back to bed for more rest. This feeling of total exhaustion is quite different from anything I've experienced. It's an all-encompassing tiredness, reaching into every extremity, every nook and cranny of my being. Even my eyelashes are feeling the effects of Salerno's surgery.

Visiting nurses and interns—mostly for my poor roomie—stop to say that it's quite normal to feel the way I do after major surgery. But their advice is suspect: they're all too young to have experienced major surgery. Only those who have been through it know for certain and with sufficient authority to explain what it's like. More and more I am convinced that someone should write a handbook on postoperative effects of major surgery presented from the patient's viewpoint and not the physician's observations. Maybe an alphabetical listing of operations, each with a thousand names and phone numbers of those who have shared the same fate. Great idea.

A few days before my transfer to hospital I received a call from California. A man I had never met heard through a mutual friend that I was going in for a by-pass. He had received his triple by-pass a year before and thought I might be interested in knowing he had survived and experienced a physical rebirth. At his expense he phoned me person-to-person in the middle of the afternoon to cheer me up, thereby providing an enormous boost to my peace of mind. I kept him on the phone much longer than simple courtesy demanded, questioning him on a variety of matters that neither doctors nor nurses seemed able to answer satisfactorily.

His physical situation, age, and first heart attack had been similar to my own, but he couldn't remain longer than one minute on the exercise bicycle without angina pain. Ninety days after the operation he started playing tennis again. Now, a year later, he was jogging three to four miles each morning before breakfast. He had even shed another wife—they tend to do everything to excess in California—and taken on another. Hadn't touched a pill or tablet for anything more severe than a headache in nearly a year. Yet we didn't talk about his first thirty days after surgery, and had I known then what I know now, I'd have had another fifteen minutes of questions to ask this kindly man.

Fortunately I have Neary to answer questions. So, I'll husband my strength for an hour or two and then go visiting. Is he experiencing the same feelings of stuffed feathers, constipation, and exhaustion? I'll find out shortly.

My stitches are beginning to itch. A wide strip of white adhesive tape hides the ones on my chest. With every breath I feel a tug of both hair and threads. I'm terrified at the thought of some nurse snatching this tape unexpectedly with a professional yank after prior assurance that "it isn't going to hurt a bit." How much longer have I got before it happens? Soon.

But the worst itching comes from that lengthy crewel-work beneath the elastic leg sock. Darby Honeyman, our ballooning angel of mercy, warned of the dangers that could develop if the leg was not given regular exercise: pooling of blood at the ankle, poor circulation, muscular atrophy. Scared hell out of me, she did. Within the hour of first consciousness after surgery I began an exercise program. So far it appears to be working. Whenever I think of it, I flex the ankle, toes, and knee joint until my chest aches. Other than an incessant itch the leg feels fine. A walk to Neary's room will be exactly the sort of thing to speed its recovery.

A slow, wobbly pace to the door. Rest against the wall outside. Dizzy, trembling, breathless. No chairs. Dreary corridor. Man across the way with head swathed in yards of bandage. Brain tumor. Victim of Victory 2. Two interns with hanging beards and stethoscopes saunter down the hall. Come by to see my roomie. He's asleep. They want to know if he's feeling better. Jesus, they're asking me?

"Isn't he dying?"

"Shhhh," one warns. "He's not to know yet. Might upset him."

True.

"How long does he have?" I gasp.

I'm wasting precious energy talking rot with the doctor. The serious one shrugs.

"Six days, six weeks—hard to say."

Neither is prepared to take odds. I lurch along the wall. First door. No Neary. Three very old women with sunken death-mask faces regard me with large, luminous eyes. Normally I'd wave. Too weak, ladies. Sorry. Next door is closed. Broom closet. Damn. His is the last door before the nurses' reception desk. Has to be. It's the only one left. The corridor is swimming, swaying like an Andean rope bridge. I clutch the wall, working my way carefully to the entrance. Neary is there, lying in bed, his face beet red. I get a weak wave.

"How about a turn along the corridor?"

Bravado. I stagger to a nearby chair and collapse. Neary

smiles. I'm not fooling anybody. Across the room seated before a sink is an old man with an electric razor working at his stubble. He's wearing pajamas and a modish dressing gown. A small circular magnifying mirror is propped against a tap. I drop him a nod. He looks vaguely familiar.

"How y'feeling now?"

"Better."

"First few days are worst," he says without taking his eyes from the mirror.

I stare. It's the same old man who came with me in the ambulance. The one Salerno had to reopen. And he's sitting up shaving? I can't believe my eyes.

"You're up and walking?"

Stupid question. Of course he is. His wife sits near the sink smiling at me. We talk. She used to be a nurse at the Victoria Hospital in London. Her husband is going to be all right now. His name is Mills. Trueman Mills. What a man.

He finishes shaving, blows the residue from the razor's head, and stands. He's my height. Broad, high forehead and bemused eyes. There's an aura of quiet power to the man. I gaze at him admiringly.

"You must have been one tough sonofabitch fifty years ago," I offer.

He smiles. "Still am."

Amen.

Neary does have feathers in his chest. He is constipated and dizzy and exhausted and "How in hell did you manage to find enough energy to make it down here?" he marvels. Which of course makes me feel much better. Nothing like a little adulation to improve the perspective. A few minutes' small chat and I wish them all *bonne chance* and stagger out the door for the long journey home.

We should all have been put in the same room. Allowed to feed from each other's emotional strengths to combat our individual weaknesses. Much too idealistic for Victory 2. Divide and conquer. Exhausted, I crawl into bed and fall asleep instantly.

Day Five. My first weigh-in. I've lost fourteen pounds. Probably peed most of it away with the diuretic pills. Helen thinks I look like a cadaver. The face that regards me gravely from the bathroom mirror is gaunt and yellow with dark raccoon rings beneath its eyes. This image, like the pain, will pass. And the pain is leaving quickly.

More walking. A little less hesitant now but still terribly weak. It is the weakness that's annoying, combined with light nausea and a feeling of dizziness. That mixture of sensations one gets after six drinks and a bad meal in a third-class restaurant with no place to throw up.

One of the nurses tried to snap the tape off my chest this morning. I fought like a tiger. If anyone is going to do it I will.

"It's my chest."

"Pooh," she sniffed.

Using her curved medical scissors, I ease the tape away from flesh, stitches, and hair, taking the better part of an hour. Virtually painless. The wound is healing nicely and looks mighty impressive. However, near the base of the incision it appears that whoever did the stitching didn't quite align the matching skin flaps, so there is now an overlap. If it heals this way I'll have a permanent ridge of raised skin at the bottom of my breastbone. A curiosity at the beach for sunbathers: "Excuse me, sir, is that a worm on your chest?"

The sock comes off twice a day for airing. My leg feels much better with it off. I decide to stop wearing it. After checking both ankles for blood pooling—and finding none—Salerno agrees.

Neary is walking at last. Seems to be about a day behind me in his recovery. I made two or three trips to his room and chided him for lying abed. It worked. Shortly after my second visit he hobbled into my room and sat down looking pained and pleased.

This evening one of the nurses actually asked if there was anything she could do for me. Helen was visiting at the time. We were speechless. Someone should have explained that this wasn't the way things were supposed to be done in Victory 2. Self-consciously she admitted that it was her first assignment to the floor and in view of the supervisory staff's attitude would in all probability be her last. To demonstrate my appreciation I asked for a glass of orange juice.

Most of the nurses I've met are dedicated humanitarians. Maybe they don't intend to become humanitarians, but that's the way things work out if they remain long in their profession. Without question, it is the nursing staff that makes or breaks a hospital's reputation. Doctors may diagnose, prescribe, examine, and operate, but it's the nurses who administer and promote a patient's sense of well-being and eventual recovery and capture the grateful hearts.

Day Six. The stitches came out of my chest today. Awkward for me to reach, so I left them for the nurse. Tweezers to lift. Sharp, needle-nosed scissors to snip. Extraordinary how swiftly the body repairs itself.

Those in my leg will remain. They are gut and designed to dissolve on their own. More difficult to sew, but leave a much less visible type of scar for those who are sensitive to stares when wearing tennis shorts. Not a problem for anyone with hairy chest and legs. In any case, the scars are guaranteed to fade within two years or double your money back.

During a short walk this afternoon it dawns on me that my angina is gone. Vanished. I stop, stunned. Normally it could be felt lurking constantly just beneath the surface, waiting for a chance to spring up and begin squeezing. No more. It's gone and taken the pain with it. Standing in the middle of the hall, I begin weeping and feel like a senile old fool. I can't help it.

The man with the broken neck sees me from his room and comes out to help, his head balancing precariously on top of its special steel and wire frame.

"Anything wrong?"

I manage an enigmatic smile and totter to the sanctuary of my bed, feeling a perfect fool.

Day Seven. Release! After final blood tests, more X-rays, and consultations Dr. Salerno decides that I am well enough to go home. He is keeping Neary for another couple of days.

There's no doubt that I'm vastly improved, but regardless of a brave physical effort and appearance, and Salerno's decision, there is still a very long way to go before recovery. On a fitness scale of one to a hundred I'm somewhere just under ten and trying hard to look like twenty.

Helen comes to get me in the early afternoon. I'm still too sore to bend and tie shoelaces or pull up my pants. Even trying to work each arm into a shirt proves to be a massive undertaking if stabs of chest pain are to be avoided.

I bid my roomie good-by. His handshake is solid and unyielding. He believes that he's getting better; he actually convinced himself that he'll recover. And why not? The pain has gone and despite his lower-body paralysis the doctors keep making positive clucking sounds when they're visiting. A deceitful scene.

His daughter is with him, a nurse from the cardiac floor of the Hotel Dieu, where I had been. Small world. She knows the hopelessness of her father's condition. It's in her eyes when she looks away. Grief and gallantry. God grant me such an understanding daughter when my time for final departure arrives.

A wheelchair comes for me. One last visit to Neary, and I'm off. There isn't a single familiar face at the nurses' reception desk for me to wish adieu. Instead, a shrewish matron adjusts her glasses and examines Helen suspiciously before checking my name off her escape list. Then I'm rolling through the honeycomb of corridors to the front door and sunshine.

Helen goes off to bring the car curbside while I sit resting on the stone steps watching the afternoon unfold. Eighty-seven steps to the car. Two major and five minor bumps on the way home that wrench my chest. I need another set of shock absorbers under my butt to flatten the uneven road. The slightest hump or depression is magnified a thousand times, like some Chinese torture machine. When we reach the house I have enough energy left to make it into the bedroom, undress, and collapse.

Day Eight. My son Peter docks in the *St. Lawrence II.* When he comes down the gangway and along the wharf looking tanned and wonderfully alive, I am standing there to greet him.

Kingston, Canada

The critical limiting factor for the success of any organ transplant is the body's rejection mechanism. Everyone is familiar with the immediate effects when a foreign substance is introduced to his body. Whether it's a heart transplant or a tiny sliver of wood, the results are the same: white blood cells rush to fight the foreign object, first trying to isolate it from spreading to other parts of the body, then encircling it in inflammatory combat, trying to destroy the intruder.

In the case of a sliver it means a sore finger until infection softens the surrounding flesh and the fragment is gently eased out of the body. In the case of a transplanted heart it means death, unless chemicals are used to combat the rejection machinery. Even then, people with heart transplants living much beyond five years are rare. Generally, some secondary infection sets in having nothing to do with the heart, and since the body's defensive mechanisms have been severely crippled from chemicals, the new infection runs rampant throughout the system.

Tissue matching for surgical transplants is an exacting science. Ideally, organs from identical twins are the most interchangeable. Or better yet, spare parts from one's own body. Yet sometimes the body fails to recognize the transplant even when it is part of its own substance. In the case of coronary by-pass operations this phenomenon happens about 12 percent of the time. On the twenty-fifth day after surgery my body's immune system began rejecting its three new by-passes.

For the first days at home I had difficulty finding a comfortable sleeping position. Our queen-sized bed had but one position: horizontal. The first night was pure hell—for Helen, too, since I kept her awake most of the night thrashing around trying to find the best and least painful arrangement. Support was the problem. In the end, using three pillows wrapped in a sheet similar to an Indonesian "Dutch wife," I was able to simulate the same horizontal back support I'd been getting from my sloping hospital bed.

Each day I walked. Very slowly and painfully at first, then gradually increasing the distances until by the end of the second week I could walk a slow mile on level ground. I was careful to choose flat terrain because the slightest sidewalk gradient left me breathless and with stars dancing in front of my eyes.

Yet something was radically wrong. I'd reached a plateau of recovery, held it for a few days, then felt myself slipping back. My two daily walks became shorter until it was all I could do just to get around the block.

Alarmed, I phoned Carol Harkness, Dr. Salerno's nurse. After discussing it with the doctor, she suggested that it might be a reaction to the Digoxin. I was to suspend all medication, get more bed rest, and stop trying to push myself so hard.

"Remember, you've had a serious operation. It will take time for your body to heal."

Tell me about it.

Within forty-eight hours, when the feelings of exhaustion and vertigo became unbearable, Helen drove me back to KGH. After an hour in emergency while an intern tried to evaluate the significance of an 80-over-95 blood pressure reading and I assured him I'd been taking no medication, a cardiologist arrived.

After a quick examination and two X-rays, he announced his findings. Pericarditis. He produced the photos and showed me the enormous shadow filling my chest cavity.

"That's my heart?"

It looked big enough to handle a bull elephant during rutting season.

"Not quite. That's your pericardium, a protective lining encasing the heart like an envelope. It's inflamed because your body is rejecting the by-passes. A watery substance collects between the heart and the pericardium, filling the sack. What you're seeing on the X-ray is a large water sack of body fluid.

Your heart is at the center, working like hell to overcome this external pressure—which is why your blood pressure is so low.

"If the pressure differential drops any lower they will insert a needle and draw off the fluid. Meanwhile, I'm putting you on Motrin to control the inflammation. We'll keep you here under observation for a few days until the situation improves."

He doesn't turn evasive when I question him, which is a good sign. Or maybe he's just a damn good actor. I'm too sick to inquire further. My head is pounding from pain.

Into a wheelchair and off to a cardiac recovery floor somewhere within the bowels of the various glass and concrete stalagmites that make up Kingston General Hospital. As long as it isn't Victory 2, I don't care. Helen brings up the rear. She must be getting to hate these places as much as I do. So far this year I've spent forty-seven days in hospital. Worse, I seem to be getting progressively sicker each time I turn up at emergency.

Cardiac recovery is in one of the newer sections. Broad, clean corridors, bright lights, slick chrome furnishings, and starched smiling nurses. I'm wheeled into a six-bed room, so already I feel better. No overhead monitors or glass-enclosed fishbowl, no hourly checks or concerned secular seclusion from other patients. Maybe I'm not that sick after all. In which case, why do I feel so rotten?

My heart is drowning slowly in its own body fluids. Bizarre. I feel as though the water levels are rising through my neck and into the brain where I'll explode eventually in a blue flash of short-circuiting cellular dipoles. And that suggestion of a needle in my chest to drain off the fluid isn't such a comforting idea either. Helen pats my hand and departs to resume the packing at home. We're leaving for Nova Scotia as soon as I'm fit to travel.

When?

Good question. The original date was set for August 1. Most unlikely now. Out of one prison and into another. There's an irony to all this, and were I in a happier frame of mind I might even be able to laugh at the situation.

I undress and climb into bed. Horizontal, my head hurts to bursting point. Sitting up feels much better. I ask the nurse to crank the bed. As she winds the handle I am introduced to the others: an incredibly frail old man who stares at me unblinkingly through his bed bars, another suffering from periods of violent fibrillation; the remaining two are asleep. They are all coronary patients. I nod politely and try for sleep. There's a secure feeling of survival lying in a hospital bed when one is sick. No matter what happens, expert help is only moments away.

In healthy middle-aged men normal blood pressure readings at rest are 135 over 80, a spread of 55 pressure points. With exercise, this spread widens. But, when the pericardium becomes inflamed and the heart muscle is placed under constant pressure from its liquid encasement, systolic pressure plummets.

Once the pressure differential narrows to a factor of less than 15 between systolic and dyastolic readings, a real danger of congestive heart failure arises: as the two pressure readings meet, there is no longer sufficient strength within the heart to overcome the pressure of the liquid. Blood no longer flows as it should. The body begins to die. The heart stops.

For the next two days my blood pressure is taken every three hours. At one point when the pressure narrows dangerously, a doctor is summoned to perform a fluid tap. Although the mechanics sound simple, in reality it is a high-risk procedure.

If the needle is inserted at the wrong angle, too deep into the chest cavity, or without the precise knowledge of how far the heart and arterial inflammation has spread, rupturing of blood vessels can occur, followed by death in mere moments. Nor is there any guarantee that the removal of liquid will correct the problem. Within a few hours the buildup can reappear exactly as before, requiring another tap.

But by the time the doctor arrives bedside and takes another reading on the sphygmomanometer the critical moment has passed, the spread widens back into the safety zone. Reprieve.

On the third day I'm feeling well enough to begin talking with my room mates. One, a pleasant-faced balding man with watery eyes, admits to a triple by-pass two years earlier and another heart attack two weeks ago. He had set up and organized the Columbia Record Club operations in Canada after the meteoric career in the United States with the parent company. The typical high-powered executive running his body on overdrive seven days a week. A hefty heart attack removed him from the game.

After his by-passes were installed a year later, he moved to the country, bought a service station to stave off boredom, and within two years was running at full speed once more. Result: a second heart attack. This time around he's scared stiff. Was the attack brought on by a narrowing in one or more of his new by-passes or had some other coronary artery become blocked? Until the doctors can do the necessary angiography he must wait in fearful speculation.

"But surely you knew this would happen again if you didn't change your lifestyle?"

I can't believe the man has a death wish. One warning is all we have a right to expect. He's had two.

He shakes his head. "I was stupid. Before I knew it, I was working fourteen hours a day seven days a week again. No more. I told my wife to put the service station up for sale."

But I can see he doesn't mean it. Not really. Not unless the doctors manage to scare him enough or the angina pains come back for a visit and decide to stay and haunt him every waking hour.

We stand looking out the tinted window at the lake. We're high above the trees, the streets, the agony of life. Sailboats puff and billow as they ride the afternoon waves. So peaceful.

"Maybe I'll just buy a boat and go sailing," he says wistfully, "while I'm still young enough to enjoy life."

And there is wisdom to his words. The secret of life is in its enjoyment. Without enjoyment, life becomes a pointless exercise of frustrations, unfulfilled ambitions, and misery.

When the late Walt Disney was at the pinnacle of success after an astonishingly productive life, a reporter asked if he was enjoying himself? "Not as much as my brother does," Disney replied. "Now there is a man who really knows how to enjoy life." His brother worked as a postman. Never a care in the world, working without stress or care. He outlived Walt.

The Motrin pills do their work. After five days a second X-ray shows that the shadow has shrunk. Not back to normal yet, but enough to let me out of hospital. This time I won't try to push myself to the limit. There's no need. No rush. No time clocks to punch or crisis meetings to attend. If I can't walk a mile this week, so what? Perhaps the week after, or week after that. I must rethink my passion for promptitude, my fetish for measuring every distance traversed. It comes from flying, I suppose—how far, how long, how high, how much gas left, how far can I glide if the motor stops? All of that is unimportant now.

Those yellow caution lights at city intersections must become signals to slow down instead of speeding up. Once it was—at least in part—a macho matter to drive the fast lane. Now, staying out of it is a survival matter. Impatience must be replaced by contentment. So obvious now. Simple to accept in theory but difficult to put into practice.

Helen drives me home. I'm not allowed behind the wheel for at least six weeks until the breastbone knits and rib cartilage damage heals. The house is a mess. Cardboard boxes line the walls in every room. In the center of the living room open trunks and suitcases stand waiting to be filled. I sit uselessly watching Helen work while depression and frustration fold in around me.

I can't lift anything heavier than a knife and fork, can't help pack the boxes or tie the stout cord around each. Worse, when visiting the supermarket I can't push the cart and have to stop between aisles to rest when my strength begins to ebb. At the checkout counter I leave everything for my one-hundred-pound wife to lug out to the car. Although she understands and accepts this absurd relationship—even with amusement—that doesn't make it any easier to endure. Such idiotic male pride.

Fortunately there is Walter Winters. Without Walter we'd be doomed. Walter is sixty and retired. When I met him he was twenty-eight and retired.

Years ago when I was a very savvy fifteen-year-old who

knew the answers to everything, but none of the right questions, my father told me that if I could make one lasting friend in life I would be achieving more than most men. At the time I thought he was full of shit. But then I thought most people were full of shit who said things I didn't understand.

During World War II Walter served in the Canadian Navy on the Murmansk run, rising eventually to command a corvette on convoy duty. We met in New Brunswick while I was finishing high school and he had begun work as a design consultant with one of the local department stores in St. John. His wife, a beautiful English war bride, ran a quaint "olde moulde tea shoppe" from their farm near the village of Hampton, while Walter commuted daily thirty miles to and from work in the battered Austin station wagon. The car had real wood siding and red leather seats. But although financial prudence forced him into the professionalism of interior design and decoration, his emotional interest remained with the tea shop at Copper Farm, as he called the place.

In those far-off days I considered Walter a wildly imprac- tical man, an adult rebel fighting the universal cause of teen-age sufferage. He seemed more of a teenager than I was, without the least concern for deadlines, the future, or the imminence of financial disaster that haunted him throughout his life. His theory was that the future would always take care of itself rather splendidly if left alone, and one should concentrate on enjoying the present.

Not a bad philosophy when I stop and reflect upon it now. We became good friends. I taught his daughter how to ride her first bicycle, witnessed his marriage fall apart, attended the auction that disposed of the remains of his beloved Copper Farm, traveled with him across the country to another life, and saw him embark on another career. Our ways parted. Two decades passed.

By accident we met again. My star was on the ascendancy, his still floating effortlessly in a happy heaven of his own making. He still had nothing, and yet he had everything. Helen adored him. For a while he operated a gift shop in a summer colony along the shores of Lake Huron, took another wife, shed her after a year, then went to England for an extended holiday to visit his ex-wife. She had contracted multiple sclerosis and Walter went to see if he could help. Extraordinary.

When he returned, I was broke and in prison. He didn't visit because he didn't want to embarrass us. Dear Walter. But the moment he learned about my heart problems, he dropped everything and drove the 350 miles from Owen Sound to Kingston to help.

After sizing up our situation, and my inability to do much of anything except get in the way while Helen was trying to arrange the packing and travel arrangements, he announced that he would be coming with us to Nova Scotia for a long-over-due holiday.

He vanished for a week to reappear with a small house trailer attached to his ancient Toyota. No charge. He had borrowed it from a friend to make the trip, thereby saving all of us the cost of motels and restaurant meals. For the first time since I'd known him, he was in better financial shape than I was—by a considerable measure. My family's finances were in a frightful state.

During the preceding week I had tried unsuccessfully for disability benefits through the government pension and unem-ployment insurance plans. No luck. A purse-lipped voice informed me in no uncertain terms that I didn't qualify for benefits because I had stopped contributing to the plans over the past few years. No, working as a pastry cook in prison didn't count as insurable work.

"But I was getting paid. It was a job. A real honest-to-God job."

"Oh no it wasn't. You're a convict!" she snapped.

Catch 22. The Canadian Penitentiary Service is not an equal-opportunity employer when it comes to disability benefits from the federal government, regardless of one's previous contributions.

I pay a last visit to Dr. Burggraf to thank him for his help and quiet insistence that I be permitted to leave prison for my convalescence after surgery. I am certain that at least twice he has saved my life by being stubborn. He gives me a letter for a cardiologist in Halifax, a colleague. Salerno is too busy saving other lives to hear my thanks. I leave them with his nurse, who promises to pass them on.

By mid-August I'm off all medication except aspirin. Two tablets each day to keep the pericarditis at bay. It works the same as Motrin. I can walk a mile—slowly—but that feeling of stuffed feathers and constant vertigo is still with me, filling my chest and brain. The movers arrive: a flurry of loading and the truck rumbles off toward the East Coast.

Our convoy follows an hour later, Walter and the girls in the Toyota, dragging the trailer; Helen and I in our sputtering Datsun with Banion the dog. Peter is away in Texas, working on a cattle ranch near Dallas for the summer—hot, heavy, dusty work in a record drought year under the supervision of one of my old flying buddies.

Two-hour segments are about all I can manage before discomfort sets in. Rest stop. Our convoy pulls off the road and parks well over on the shoulder. I ease myself out of the front seat and lean against the side of the car, waiting for my vertigo to subside. The steady driving motion brings nausea and light dizziness. What would happen in an airplane? The thought makes me ill. Six weeks since the operation and I'm still terribly weak and plagued by chest pains and motion sickness. Some may be able to recover from the ordeal in thirty days, as the doctors claim, but obviously I'm not one of them. How long then?

Before leaving Kingston I checked with Neary and was comforted to learn that he still found trouble climbing stairs or walking for longer than fifteen minutes. No nausea or dizziness though: he's been spared that annoyance. Lucky man. Maybe this ailment is peculiar to my recovery. Why? When I questioned Burggraf he didn't seem to have any answers, but assured me that it would pass. How does he know?

Cars and trucks swhoosh past on the highway. Following them with my eyes increases the vertigo and nausea. Don't look. Helen stands talking to Walter. They appear as two people viewed through the wrong end of a telescope. My eyes are playing little tricks and relaying the wrong dimensions to my brain. A game. I want to throw up.

The girls gambol with Banion along the grassy slopes, searching for wildflowers and four-leaf clovers. Our dog, still a puppy really, is a blond-haired mutt with an enormous white powder-puff tail that swishes majestically with every step. He's stupid, unruly, undisciplined, and a complete coward. We adore him. Surprisingly, he travels well, sleeping contentedly in the back of the station wagon until Helen stops; then he's all bark and excitement for whatever action is going.

Last winter one of the Frontenac inmates found him abandoned in a rock quarry at the edge of the prison's property and brought him back to camp. For a while he remained in the basement, fed and petted by every passing con until the warden, a cat lover, ordered him off the premises. The girls carried him home as a present from the man who found him. He became our terrified watchdog and in at least two instances prevented the house from being broken into by marauding teenagers. Despite his appalling lack of brains he is the prettiest-looking dog I've seen for some time.

Within minutes my equilibrium returns, the nausea subsides. During her three pregnancies Helen suffered horribly from nausea. She understands my problem better than anyone.

"Ready?" Walter asks.

I'd like to stretch out on the grass and let the rest of this day laze past. Can't be done. Convoys move only as fast as the slowest vessel. I'm holding up the war.

"Let's go."

Our next stop is Upper Canada Village. Antiquity on the banks of the St. Lawrence River, where carefully reconstructed shops and houses, dusty streets carefully swept, actors and actresses dressed in period costumes, reflect what once was and will never be again. It's all too perfect for my liking, like a TV period piece. Missing are the smells of fresh horse dung, creak, squeak, and jingle of leather harness, and the real salty glisten of human sweat worn as a fact of human toil.

Walter and I lie on the grass under a shade tree while Helen takes the girls on tour of the place. Banion curls into a ball at the end of his chain and stares at me morosely. It's a clear blue-green day with yellow shadows filtering through the branches to splay across the grass.

"Ever think about dying, Walter?"

"Constantly. Why?"

"Just wondering."

He props himself on one elbow and yanks a grass stem to chew from the stubble carpet.

"I figure that if I can get through my sixties without getting hit by heart problems or cancer, every year after that is a bonus. How about you?"

He has twelve years on me. Right now I feel closer to eighty than fifty. Walter is the youngster, I'm the old man. Where the hell have my strength and energy gone? Will they ever return again?

"I figured everything after July second was a bonus. I'm still living on borrowed time."

He examines me quizzically. "You look a lot better than you did a week ago. Truly. I'm not bullshitting you. You do. You're getting better. It takes time."

Then why do I feel so rotten? My angina has been cured at what price? Feel weak and dizzy and ill or feel that terrifying clutch of angina. Take your pick. You can't have it both ways. Them's the rules.

Why?

Neither Burggraf nor Salerno said a thing about any physical toll that would have to be paid for coronary salvation: "Oh, by the way, Foster—should have mentioned it earlier— your body will be wrecked for a while after surgery. Fifty percent of patients never return to normal active lives again—ever. But then again, maybe you'll confound the odds and turn out to be one of the lucky ones. Ha-ha!"

And Walter tells me that I look better. I manage a smile.

"You're a terrible liar. I know I look like hell. But thanks anyway."

Night in a picturesque trailer park on the Quebec border, among towering trees and swarms of high rpm mosquitoes. Helen, the girls, and I bed down in the trailer while Walter snuggles into a sleeping bag inside the station wagon, feet protruding from the open door. Sleep is instantaneous.

Four days later we arrive in Halifax to begin searching for a new home, new schools, new friends, a new life. A moment of rebirth. I'm beginning to feel a bit better.

Halifax, Canada

Christmas Day, 1980

A cold white day with fresh snow piled high on rooftops, and overhead a huge bright sun without a thimbleful of warmth for cheeks, noses, toes, or fingers. Joy to the world!

The attendants pick their way carefully through the drifts to the ambulance and slide me and the stretcher inside. Thirteen minutes to Victoria Hospital. Another Victoria Hospital. They sprout like mushrooms from coast to coast, *a mari usque ad mare*. Oxygen mask. Anxious attendant. Wheeping siren. *Deja vu*.

Helen follows in the station wagon. The advantage of living in Halifax is that everything's so close at hand. Fifteen minutes maximum from anywhere to everywhere. Twenty minutes in rush hour. No rush on Christmas Day. The best of all days for a hospital emergency. Even lacerated drunks observe a Christmas truce.

My symptoms are familiar: chest pains, nausea, shortness of breath, general weakness. Is it another heart attack?

I had been out walking the dog. Once around the block for exercise in the bitterly cold air. Cold air plays hell with angina sufferers. I know. I remember. Something hit me. A terrible weakness in the legs and arms. The dog dragged me home. With the last dregs of strength I staggered into the house and collapsed, soaked in perspiration and the certainty of my approaching demise.

But now, in the braying ambulance, I realize that it doesn't feel exactly like the heart attack in Kingston, and the closer we get to hospital the more I feel like a medical fraud. I don't need the oxygen and my chest pains have diminished considerably since Helen phoned the hospital.

Nonetheless, upon arrival I'm wheeled into cardiac emergency and quickly given the complete treatment. Helen wears that strained, tight look I've come to recognize. By the time a young intern—why are they always so young?—confronts me with the statistical evidence of my physical deceit, I'm well enough to get up and go home mumbling apologies for being such a bloody fool. Instead, I try to look suitably subdued.

"Blood pressure, ECG, temperature, all normal. The lab is closed for the holiday, so we won't have the results on your blood for a few days. You had a by-pass operation?"

"Six months ago."

"Any postoperative complications?"

There's that word again: complications. The unforeseen. The unpredictable. The dirty word.

"Pericarditis."

He nods and makes a note on his file. I could tell him how from September to November I went steadily downhill from nausea, vertigo, and general weakness until finally, when no longer capable of getting out of bed, I became convinced that I was dying. It was then that Helen suggested I stop taking pills—including the aspirin—and see what would happen.

What happened was that I started at once to get better. My problem stemmed from an allergy to aspirin. At one time I could devour a dozen of the little white tablets with no ill effects. But after Kingston something must have happened to my metabolism. Aspirin joined penicillin as another of my allergies. When I asked my new family doctor to explain, he couldn't.

Mystery. Heal thyself.

Once I was well enough to begin walking again, I decided to embark on a carefully controlled program of self-experimentation to learn what else might cause problems. I discovered that medically prescribed "safe" pills such as Motrin, Anacin, Tylenol, and codeine-based cough syrups or headache tablets produced virtually the same results of vertigo, nausea, and general malaise. For some undefined reason my body would no longer tolerate chemical intrusions.

I could explain all this to the intern but it might test his credulity, and certainly my own credibility. A single postoperative complication of pericarditis sounds much less bizarre than the facts.

In these last months I've become a walking encyclopedia of medical knowledge, techniques, and buzz words. All doctors acquire their power from books and experience. No reason why I couldn't do the same. And the more I learn, the more I realize how much is unknown. Specific ailments requiring the proper dosages of drugs, possible side effects, healing time, and suggested alternatives if the first attempt fails.

But nonspecific ailments are different. Only familiarity with symptoms can provide a theory for each problem. But there are no guarantees that the local physician can recognize any but the most obvious of symptoms or connect them to a specific ailment. How many general practitioners in North America recognize a diver's bends, malaria, or dengue fever on sight? Precious few, I'd be willing to bet.

My symptoms are nonspecific. This worries the young intern. Is the by-pass acting up? Am I suffering from psychosomatic delusions? Maybe I'm one of those hospital freaks who loves taking up bed space. What to do?

"I think we should keep you under observation a few days, just in case a problem develops."

When in doubt, check the patient into hospital—the wait-and-see approach. Here we go again.

While Helen fills in the forms at Admissions, I am wheeled off to Cardiac Care. Like the Hotel Dieu in Kingston, it is on the fourth floor of a new annex: "Centennial," which means that it was built circa 1967.

The fishbowl has six beds in one room, a monitor over every patient's head. It is impossible to watch one's own recordings because of the angle at which the unit is placed above the bed, but everyone else in the room can engage in electronic voyeurism.

There are no introductions. A few cheery hellos from the other older men as I'm bedded down and stabbed in quick succession with needles: in the stomach for a heparin injection, in the wrist for an I.V. connection, and in the forearm for more blood. The doctor won't be in until much later.

"It's Christmas, you know."

Sensible fellow. Only the direst emergency should recall a doctor on Christmas Day.

A nurse administers Inderal, Anturan, and a Valium to relax me. I check the tablets. Only twenty milligrams of Inderal.

"Don't go over forty milligrams or my heart will stop," I caution.

"Right. Forty milligrams. Got it."

She takes my pulse, temperature, and blood pressure while I lie watching a monitor on the other wall. Incredible. The man across the way is asleep. His heart stops beating for three- or four-second intervals at irregular times, then thumps quickly to catch up. Is this normal? It doesn't appear to bother the nurse. She's a frumpy-looking farm girl with soft, fat fingers and a patient disposition. Someone has to work on Christmas Day.

In the far corner an old fisherman climbs out of bed, balances on one leg and announces in a loud voice that it's time he "got goin'. Can't be layin' about here all day."

The nurses guide him gently back to bed and settle him under the covers. My farm girl explains that the old man is ninety-two and still very active. He lost a foot in an accident years ago. To keep him from escaping they have taken away his prosthesis. Once he managed to make it all the way down to the main entrance before getting nabbed in the lobby.

"Poor man. Now his heart is failing along with his mind. Don't you think old age is sad?" she asks me quietly.

Indeed I do.

Ego boosting on Christmas Day. Compared with the other old crocks, I'm a spring chicken and she recognizes it. God rest ye, merrie gentlemen!

Helen drops by for a minute before rushing away to a Christmas dinner with the children at her parents' table. She'll bring my toothbrush, pajamas, and shaving gear later.

"Give my apologies. I'll try to make it next year."

Always assuming I'm around to make it next year. My in-laws have reached their eighties in better shape than I am now. How the hell did they do it? Was it lack of stress or abundant contentment? Magic formula for longevity: one happy man, one happy woman. Mix gently over a lifetime of love, mutual admiration and understanding, a dash of excitement, two pinches of sorrow, simmer gently until ready to serve.

My father died of cancer in his early sixties. He and my father-in-law were first cousins, born within sixty days of each other, attended the same schools, graduated from university, and rose eventually to the top of their professions. Strange. My affable, unflappable father-in-law I'm certain will last well into his nineties. Hopefully, my children will inherit some of the important genes from his side of our family, thereby sparing them from cancer and heart disease.

I doze through the afternoon, afloat on a Valium cloud of faint indifference. Helen reaches me briefly during evening visiting hours. Incoherent discussion about incomprehensible subjects. I can't remember her leaving or if she brought the things I asked for.

More pills before bedtime. I'm too groggy to check them. Why are they giving me so many pills? Do they know what they're doing? Does anyone nowadays? Where have all the doctors gone? Who is managing the store—that peach-faced intern down at emergency? As I drift into sleep there is a bright feeling of foreboding. A flashing neon against the dark horizon. But I'm too far away to read the words.

Near four in the morning I'm awakened by an anxious-faced nurse.

"We're operating on you."

"You are?"

Warning bells jangle in my brain. Instantly I'm awake and ready to protest. What the hell is she talking about? If they want to operate on me at this hour, shouldn't someone check with my cardiologist or my family doctor—or my wife?

"Your heart keeps stopping. The periods between pauses are getting shorter and we're afraid it might stop altogether. So the doctor is coming in to give you a pacemaker, just to be on the safe side."

Wonderful. The safe side of what?

I feel my pulse. It's erratic, long pauses, slow beat. She's right. Something's wrong. So there is a problem after all and it wasn't just imagination that my legs felt weak yesterday. I have a flash of terror momentarily, then phlegmatic acceptance of the inevitable.

The room is very quiet, bathed in dim night light. Like some irregular chorus line badly in need of rehearsal, the eerie green blips on each monitor dance along the wall above the beds The old crocks are sleeping. Even the fisherman appears to be resting—or faking, waiting for his next opening to escape.

Attendants arrive, lift me onto an operating room gurney, and wheel me out of the fishbowl. They're running, almost. Urgency in their actions. Along the corridors, in and out of an elevator. Down deserted hallways. Silence except for the rush of rubber wheels. They don't want me to talk.

Jesus, it must be serious.

A nurse and a doctor are scrubbing up in the operating room. Both look as if they had been awakened recently from a sound sleep. How does one find an operating surgeon at four in the morning on Boxing Day? "Hello, doctor? We have a Coronary Care patient with a heart that keeps stopping. Question is, should we let him succumb or do you want to get up, pull on your woollies, and drive over to give him a pacemaker? No hurry. He probably has another ten or fifteen minutes."

They glance at me with interest.

"How y'feeling?" The doctor dries his hands.

"Sleepy."

"Me too."

His accent is English public school with a light Midlands undertone. I apologize for rousting him out of bed at such a frightful hour. His nurse, too.

"Any idea why my heart is acting up?"

"Haven't the vaguest," he says affably in a tone that somehow manages to imply he doesn't do shirts or windows either. It's the approved professional position of ignorance as to cause, claiming only knowledge necessary for salvation. I can recognize the play.

The nurse lifts the shirty, spreads my legs, drapes my

privates, and begins shaving the hair above the femoral artery with a very dry razor.

When the flesh is scraped bare, she swabs the area liberally with orange Mercresin antiseptic. The stuff smells like the Friar's Balsam that my mother made me inhale as a boy for chest colds. It didn't work worth a damn, but the odor remained fixed in my memory.

The doctor slips a long needle into the inside of my thigh near the groin.

"Zylocain," he mutters. "Local anesthetic. Not to worry."

The entry procedure is the same as for an angiogram. This hospital's surgeons advocate entrance through the femoral artery to reach the heart.

"Causes fewer problems. Much easier approach," the doctor claims as he slices into the surface skin.

At Kingston General this would be considered heresy. Different hospital, different approach. Which one is correct? Probably both. The end result is the same.

A long catheter with two small wires protruding from its end is slipped into the artery and fed up into my heart. Very slowly the doctor manipulates the wires through the catheter, extending them until they appear on the TV monitor like a pair of weaving grasshopper's antennae.

Once the wires are nestled into position against the heart muscle, the catheter is taped into place at the entry point.

"You're going to leave it in?"

Open artery, waving wires, adhesive tape. The whole business strikes me as a bit crude.

"Temporary installation. Not to worry."

But just the same I do.

The two exposed wires coming out of my groin are attached to a small metal battery pack. This pack, no larger than a cigarette package, is equipped with a numbered dial on which any heartbeat-per-minute demand can be set.

A pacemaker's function is, not to provide continuous electrical impulses for the heart, but rather to help when the heart fails to maintain its normal rhythm. At a setting of 55, electrical impulses will prevent the heart rate from dropping below 55 beats a minute. Or, should the heart hesitate for a fraction of a second to beat on cue, a light stimulus by the pacemaker will jog its muscular memory. It is a marvel of medical science.

"Let's check it out," the doctor says.

He twists the dial slowly past 50. I wait. What is supposed to happen? Then, suddenly, I feel it. My heart begins to beat faster, faster, until he has it racing up at 100 beats a minute. Is there such a thing as a runaway pacemaker?

He backs it down. The pace slows.

"Working fine," he announces. "I'll set it at fifty-five."

I thank him for his help and apologize again for getting him out of bed. He gives his rubber gloves a snap.

"Not to worry."

Back in the fishbowl, everyone is still asleep, including the old fisherman. My battery pack is hung on an I.V. support pole at the end of the bed, its wires trailing under the bedclothes.

"Try and get some sleep," the anxious-faced nurse advises.

But I'm not tired. I ask for a Valium. Can't be done. I'm not allowed to have any more pills until the senior resident has seen me.

Why? Have they given me too many already? Or the wrong type? But the nurse refuses to be drawn into any discussion covering these matters. Everything is to be left for the senior resident to explain.

Helen comes later in the day. Someone phoned her during breakfast, informing her about my pacemaker. After the fact? They didn't want to worry her by phoning earlier, is the somewhat illogical explanation. We discuss the situation gravely. All very fishy.

Toward evening I begin to feel most peculiar. A combination of chest tightness and wildly flipping heartbeats. A nurse studies my monitor, then goes off to get help. The old boy across the room studies my monitor. An intern and another nurse arrive to study my monitor. Everyone gets to study my goddamn monitor but me.

While the experts are all out in the hall discussing the matter *sotto voce*, I reach up and unhook the battery pack, twisting the dial around to off. My problems are solved. Instantaneously. So there is such a thing as a runaway monitor! I return it to the pole and lie back, watching the corridor discussions.

They decide on an X-ray. When in doubt get an X-ray. Soon a machine appears towing a small female driver with red hair and enormous freckles. "Sit up! Hold this! Sit still! Deep breath! Hold it! Gotcha!" And she's towed out to develop the results.

Later, after studying the pictures, no one is any the wiser, but since my monitor shows no further irregularities, it's decided that the crisis has passed. I get a good night's sleep.

In the morning after breakfast the senior resident visits: an older man with gray hair and wise eyes focused behind steel-rimmed no-nonsense spectacles. The first thing he does after glancing at my X-ray is reach under the covers and remove the catheter and pacemaker, then press the artery to seal.

"Felt strange, did it?"

"Very."

"I'm not surprised. It was sitting in the wrong position."

"I turned it off last night."

"So I see," he smiles. "Did you know you have a reaction to Inderal?"

"Above forty milligrams."

"You should have told someone."

"I did."

Two mistakes in less than twenty-four hours. Hospitals are dangerous places. People are dying in them every day. Even the healthy are not exempt.

My blood tests are negative. There was no heart attack, but I'm kept in hospital another week . . . just in case.

On the second day of the new year, armed with two brand-new prescriptions for more pills, I am released finally to return home.

My first chore, even before unpacking my things, is a visit

to the bathroom medicine cabinet. Plastic containers of Valium, Motrin, codeine, Inderal, Anturan, Digoxin, Tylenol, Anacin, and aspirin are emptied into the toilet. Last of all, I tear the new prescriptions into tiny pieces, then flush everything away. Forever.

Epilogue
Halifax, Canada
2 August 1982

There are limitations that are painful to accept emotionally. The vertigo is still with me in varying degrees of nauseous intensity. Lengthy car rides, air travel, sail boating, or prolonged physical exertion must be approached with caution and the expectation of illness. Did something happen while I was on the heart-lung machine to cause this neurological imbalance? I'll never know.

I do know that I shall never fly again or run or swim. Simple pleasures such as tennis, soccer, or playing catch or tossing a frisbee with my children are now forbidden lest the vertigo level me for a day or two. Such a silly weakness.

Worse, lifting any weight over twenty pounds hurts my chest and induces symptoms similar to the onslaught of a coronary. For over a year I lived with the fear that this is what it was, that life must be spent in the twilight, waiting for the inevitable.

Quite by chance I discovered that, in one out of every hundred by-pass operations, the rib cartilage anchored at the sternum never heals properly. Surgeons don't like to talk about it.

Instead of a normal horizontal flexing by the ribs with each breath, a vertical flex exists within the damaged cartilage when physical strain is placed on the arms or shoulders. Lifting or carrying heavy loads causes severe, nearly breathless pain that mimics angina and a coronary attack.

Prescribed medication is Motrin or aspirin. No thanks. I'll manage.

But I can walk. And do. Miles. Every day, in all types of weather, in all seasons. At least three fast-paced miles, sometimes as much as five, before the vertigo gets me. Walking has become a habit.

Periodically, and with a wry smile, I read and hear of how the latest internationally known by-pass recipient is up and about feeling "just great" a few short weeks after his operation.

Horseshit. I know better. A few might make the unusual recovery, but from my experience in talking to other members of our club, the majority are like me. They hurt for a long, long time.

It took me a year to get over the effects of the operation, to heal, regain my strength, and understand the variation of different new pains that came and went throughout the recovery period. Another six months were needed to come to terms with the realities of my new physical limitations.

Was it worth it? Faced with the same choice, would I do it all over again?

You bet.

The alternative is so permanent.

There are so many additional bonuses. I have recovered that awareness of life remembered as a boy when sights and sounds bring pleasure instead of the sophistication of adult indifference. My pace of life has changed. There's no longer any rush because nothing is really so important that it can't wait an extra hour or day—or week. I refuse to be rushed, to rejoin the old stale game, and I pity the survivors who still haven't discovered the difference between necessity and choice.

Possibly it is the maritime atmosphere: slow-moving like the tides, proud parochial values that judge a man's worth by his stance against adversity. Values forgotten long ago by the denizens of our business and bureaucratic jungles.

I have come home.

Evening enfolds my senses. Damp rich smell of ocean mists pooling in the garlands of city streetlights. From the harbor a basso foghorn grumbles disconsolately. There is a magic in every moment.

Far out on the eastern Atlantic the second half of my century dawns in golden promise. For a while longer at least, I do not feel the night coming down.